Determinants of micronutrient status, DDT residues and
pregnancy outcomes: cross-sectional studies in pregnant
and post partum women from Maela refugee camp,
North-Western Thailand

Dissertation zur Erlangung des Doktorgrades
der Naturwissenschaften (Dr. rer. nat.)

Fakultät Naturwissenschaften
Universität Hohenheim

Institut für Biologische Chemie und Ernährungswissenschaften

vorgelegt von

Wolfgang Stütz

aus *Weingarten*

2009

Bibliografische Information der Deutschen Nationalbibliothek

Die Deutsche Nationalbibliothek verzeichnet diese Publikation in der
Deutschen Nationalbibliografie; detaillierte bibliografische Daten sind
im Internet über http://dnb.d-nb.de abrufbar.

ISBN 978-3-8325-2651-1

D100

Logos Verlag Berlin GmbH
Comeniushof, Gubener Str. 47,
10243 Berlin
Tel.: +49 (0)30 42 85 10 90
Fax: +49 (0)30 42 85 10 92
INTERNET: http://www.logos-verlag.de

Dekan: Prof. Dr. Heinz Breer

1. berichtende Person: Prof. Dr. H.K. Biesalski
2. berichtende Person: Prof. Dr. T. Grune

Eingereicht am: 19. Dezember 2009

Die vorliegende Arbeit wurde am 17.05.2010 von der Fakultät Naturwissenschaften der Universität Hohenheim als „Dissertation zur Erlangung des Doktorgrades der Naturwissenschaften" angenommen.

Vortrag und mündliche Prüfung am: 19. Juli 2010

Prüfer im Kolloquium

1. Prof. Dr. med. H.K. Biesalski (Betreuer)
2. Prof. Dr. med. T. Grune
3. Prof. Dr. med. H.G. Classen

Maela camp

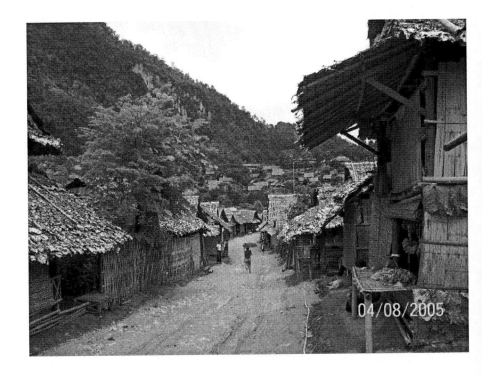

Supervisors

Prof. Dr. med. Hans Konrad Biesalski
Director of the Institute of Biological Chemistry and Nutrition,
University of Hohenheim

Prof. Dr. med. François Henry Nosten
Director of the Shoklo Malaria Research Unit, Mae Sot, Thailand
Mahidol Oxford University Research Unit

Table of contents

Summary

Rationale: Micronutrient malnutrition remains prevalent in the displaced population on the north-western border of Thailand. Deficiency of thiamine and vitamin A as well as high prevalence of anaemia were documented in pregnant and postpartum women of Maela refugee camp (pop: 45 000). Food rations provided by charities are adequate in energy and protein but low in micronutrient content. During antenatal care pregnant and lactating women receive additional food and supplements of thiamine, folic acid and ferrous sulphate. In July 2004 whole wheat flour fortified with vitamins and minerals was introduced to the whole population in Maela.

DDT was sprayed as an insecticide to control malaria until 2000. Its residues may interact with micronutrients and may affect pregnancy outcomes.

Objectives: To examine effects of antenatal iron and micronutrient supplementation and of introduced micronutrient enriched flour (MEF) on biochemical status of iron and micronutrients during pregnancy and in post partum; to elucidate the implication by micronutrients and DDT on pregnancy outcomes.

Methods: Two cross-sectional and follow-up studies among pregnant (n>1000, 1st to 3rd trimester) and breast-feeding (n>600, at week 12 post partum) women between 2004 and 2007 for the determination of iron status (serum ferritin, soluble transferrin receptor), whole blood thiamine, serum micronutrients (retinol, α-tocopherol, β-carotene, zinc, copper) and DDT residues and of iron, thiamine, micronutrient and DDT levels in breast milk.

All the pregnant women were followed to assess pregnancy outcomes (gestational age, birth weight, infant length, head- and arm circumference) and their relationship with blood micronutrients and DDT residues during pregnancy.

Results: Iron status, serum retinol, zinc, and β-carotene decreased during pregnancy. Retinol and zinc were higher whereas iron status and β-carotene were significantly lower in post partum than in early pregnancy. Whole blood thiamine increased with the number of weeks the supplement was provided and was still high at 12 weeks post partum. Serum α-tocopherol, copper and DDT residues during pregnancy increased concurrently with cholesterol and triglycerides and were significantly lower in post partum. Milk levels of iron, thiamine, micronutrients except zinc and DDT were positively correlated to their respective blood levels in post partum. Markers for iron status indicated a decrease of iron stores and a high prevalence of iron deficiency anemia (one of 3 women) in late pregnancy despite high doses of provided ferrous sulphate. In addition the prevalence of zinc deficiency was notably high in both pregnant and breast-feeding women. The introduction of micronutrient enriched flour (MEF) had a significant positive impact on zinc and iron status: post partum women (PP1) who were initially provided with the MEF had significantly higher serum zinc and an improved iron status by means of lower soluble transferrin receptor (sTfR) and higher breast-milk iron compared to those post partum women (PP) who never received the flour; two years later serum zinc in each trimester of pregnancy and serum zinc and iron status (sTfR) in post partum were significantly higher than before the introduction of MEF.

DDT residues were mainly predicted by the years the women had been resident in Thailand rather than Burma; the number of former breast-fed children reduced the amount of DDT in serum and breast milk. Four to six years after the last DDT residual house spraying the previously described interactions between DDT's residues and vitamin A in serum of pregnant women were no longer obvious.

Gestational age, mother's weight and parity were the predominant determinants of pregnancy outcomes. Low gestational age at delivery, low maternal weight, nulliparity, smoking and female gender increased the risk of low birth weight (<2500 grams). Overall mean infant's birth weight and length, gestational age at outcome, mother's weight and serum α-tocopherol and zinc increased whereas DDT residues significantly decreased during the two years study period. Multivariate regression analysis revealed that serum fat adjusted α-tocopherol was a significant positive predictor whereas high iron storage, highest hematocrit levels, fat adjusted DDT residues, as well as elevated α-1 glycoprotein (AGP >1g/L - indicating infections) during pregnancy were significant negative predictors of mean birth weight. Hematocrit >37.5%, iron storage, serum fat adjusted DDT, and AGP >1g/L were also significantly inversely related to infant's arm circumference. Whole blood thiamine per volume and per hemoglobin had a significant positive impact on infant's length. Serum β-carotene and α-tocopherol were positively whereas serum retinol, DDT and AGP >1g/L were negatively associated with newborn's head circumference.

2

Conclusion: Thiamine status following supplementation during pregnancy results in adequate blood concentrations in pregnant and post-partum women and reflects good compliance to supplementation. On the contrary the high prevalence of iron deficiency despite the provision of ferrous sulphate suggests inadequate dietary sources of iron and a low acceptance to iron supplements. An improvement of compliance compared to iron supplements is eligible. MEF showed a sustainable positive effect on zinc and iron status in both pregnant and lactating women. The provision of zinc supplements and the enrichment of already well accepted food such as fish paste would be further promising measures to reduce the prevalence of zinc and iron deficiency. Vitamin A deficiency is not a severe public health problem in Maela and serum retinol was no longer obviously confounded by DDT residues.

Blood levels of α-tocopherol, β-carotene and thiamine di-phosphate during pregnancy were positively whereas high iron status, highest hematocrit, elevated AGP and DDT residues were found to be negatively associated with newborn's weight and size parameters. Iron status and micronutrient levels in pregnancy may have direct effects or may be markers for other predictors of these pregnancy outcomes. High iron status, high serum retinol and highest hematocrit levels, particular in 3rd trimester, could reflect insufficient hemodilution and therefore reduced placental blood flow and fetal development. Higher α-tocopherol might be simply the consequence of an increased intake of vegetable oil or might reflect a well-balanced antioxidant status. The positive impact by thiamine on foetal growth regarding length is an important finding which identified thiamine supplements as an effective intervention to increase newborn length in a population having one third of pregnant women <150 cm of height. The impact by in utero exposure to DDT on birth weight even though being significant was small. DDT effects on pregnancy outcomes and micronutrient levels might be more obvious in endemic malaria areas where it is actually in regular use for indoor residual spraying but need to be carefully assessed in context to its efficiency in controlling malaria and to disease burden in high-transmission areas.

Zusammenfassung

Rationale: Die Versorgung mit Mikronährstoffen in den Flüchtlingslagern entlang der nordwestlichen Grenze Thailands ist unzureichend. Im Maela camp, der bis heute größten Siedlung mit Flüchtlingen (45000 Einwohner) aus dem benachbarten Burma stellen Thiamin- und Vitamin A Mangel sowie Anämie während als auch nach der Schwangerschaft ein ständiges Probem dar. Die von Wohlfahrtsstiftungen bereitgestellten Lebensmittelrationen liefern ausreichend Energie und Proteine doch zuwenig an lebensnotwendigen Mikronährstoffen. Schwangere und stillende Frauen erhalten bei der Betreuung in den Kliniken zusätzliche Lebensmittelrationen sowie Supplemente an Thiamin, Folsäure, und Eisensulfat. Im Juli 2004 wurde ein mit Vitaminen und Spurenelementen angereichertes Mehl als ergänzendes Nahrungsmittel für die in Maela lebende Bevölkerung eingeführt. DDT wurde hier bis zum Jahre 2000 als Insektizid zur Kontrolle von Malaria eingesetzt. Die daraus resultierenden Rückstände könnten mit Mikronährstoffen interagieren sowie einen schädlichen Einfluß auf den Schwangerschaftsverlauf ausüben.

Studienziele: Bewertung des Einflußes von Eisen- und Mikronährstoffsupplementen und Mikronährstoff angereichertem Mehl auf den Eisen- und Mikronährstoffstatus in der Schwangerschaft und in post partum; Bedeutung und Konsequenz der Mikronährstoffe und DDT Rückstände für die fötale Entwicklung und den Erfolg der Schwangerschaft.

Methoden: Zwischen 2004 und 2007 wurden zwei Querschnitts- und follow-up Studien mit schwangeren (n>1000, 1-3. Trimenon) und stillenden Frauen (n>600, in Woche 12 post partum) zur Bewertung des Eisenstatus (Serum ferritin, Transferrin Rezeptor) und zur Bestimmung von Thiamin im Vollblut, Mikronährstoffen (Retinol, α-Tocopherol, β-Carotin, Zink, Kupfer) und DDT Rückständen im Serum sowie von Eisen, Thiamin, Mikronährstoffen und DDT in der Frauenmilch durchgeführt.
Als funktionelle Indikatoren für den Ernährungsstatus und Verlauf der Schwangerschaften wurden Alter, Gewicht, Größe sowie Kopf- und Armumfang der Neugeborenen und deren Relation zu den gemessenen Mikronährstoffen und DDT Rückständen im Blut während der Schwangerschaft bewertet.

Ergebnisse: Der Eisenstatus sowie Retinol, Zink und β-Carotene im Serum nahmen mit zunehmender Schwangerschaftswoche ab. In der 12. Woche post partum waren Retinol und Zink höher, jedoch β-Carotene und der Eisenstatus signifikant niedriger als im ersten Trimester der Schwangerschaft. Thiamin im Vollblut nahm mit Anzahl der Wochen an ausgegebenen Supplementen zu und war nachhaltig hoch in post partum. In der Schwangerschaft nahmen α-Tocopherol, Kupfer und DDT Rückstände im Serum gleichzeitig mit Cholesterol und Triglyzeriden kontinuierlich zu und waren signifikant niedriger in post partum. Die Konzentrationen an Eisen, Thiamin, DDT und der Mikronährstoffe in der Milch mit Ausnahme von Zink korrelierten positiv mit den entsprechenden Blutwerten in post partum. Trotz höchster Dosen ausgegebenem Eisensulfats zeigten Indikatoren für den Eisenstatus eine hohe Prävalenz an leeren Speichern sowie Eisenmangelanämie (eine von drei Frauen) im dritten Trimenon. Zudem war der Anteil an schwangeren und stillenden Frauen mit Zinkmangel bemerkenswert hoch. Mit Einführung des ‚Mikronährstoff angereicherten Mehles' (MAM) zeigte sich eine signifikante Verbesserung des Zink- und Eisenstatus: Frauen in post partum welche während der Stillphase mit MAM versorgt wurden hatten signifikant höheres Serum Zink und einen verbesserten Eisenstatus (niedrigere Transferrin Rezeptor Werte im Serum und höhere Eisenkonzentrationen in der Milch) als vergleichbare Frauen in post partum welche das Mehl noch nicht erhielten. Zwei Jahre später waren Serum Zink in der Schwangerschaft sowie Serum Zink und Eisenstatus in post partum signifikant höher als vor der Einführung des MAM.

Die Menge an DDT Rückstände erklärten sich in der Hauptsache über die Aufenthaltszeit in Thailand und Anzahl bereits zuvor gestillter Kinder: DDT und Metaboliten im Serum und der Frauenmilch nahmen mit der Anzahl der Jahre im Maela camp oder in Thailand lebend signifikant zu; dagegen nahmen die Rückstandsmengen mit der Anzahl der Stillmonate bzw. bereits gestillter Kinder signifikant ab. Vier bis sechs Jahre nach dem letzten DDT Einsatz in den Häusern im Maela camp war die zuvor in Vorstudien beschriebene Wechselwirkung zwischen DDT Rückständen und Serum Vitamin A in der Schwangerschaft nicht mehr offensichtlich.

Die ausschlaggebenden Faktoren für eine erfolgreiche Schwangerschaft waren vor allem Schwangerschaftsdauer sowie das Gewicht und die Parität der Mutter. Frühgeburten, niedriges Gewicht der Mutter, Rauchen, das erstgeborene Kind und weibliches Geschlecht des Neugeborenen waren mit einem Risiko für ein zu niedriges Geburtsgewicht (<2500 Gramm) oder intrauterine Wachstumsstörungen assoziiert. Insgesamt nahmen über die Studienzeit von mehr als 2 Jahren das Gewicht und die Größe der Neugeborenen, das Schwangerschaftsalter am Tag der Entbindung, und das Gewicht sowie α-Tocopherol und Zink im Serum der Mütter signifikant zu; DDT Rückstände nahmen im gleichen Zeitraum signifikant ab.

Multivariate Regressionsanalysen zeigten Serumfett-korrigiertes α-Tocopherol in der Schwangerschaft als einen signifikant positiven Prädiktor für das Geburtsgewicht. Dagegen zeigten hohe Eisenspeicher, höchste Hämatokritwerte, fettkorrigierte DDT-konzentrationen und ein erhöhtes α-1 Glykoprotein (AGP, Marker für Infektionen) einen signifikant negativen Einfluss auf das Gewicht und den Armumfang der Neugeborenen. Thiamin im Vollblut und korrigiert nach Hämoglobinwerten hatte einen signifikant positiven Einfluss auf die Geburtsgröße der Kinder. Serum β-Carotene und a-Tocopherol in der Schwangerschaft zeigten einen signifikant positiven Einfluss auf den Kopfumfang; Serum Retinol, DDT und erhöhtes AGP waren negativ mit dem Kopfumfang der Neugeborenen assoziiert.

Schlussfolgerung: Der Thiaminstatus gemessen an Thiaminkonzentrationen im Blut war mehr als zufriedenstellend und spiegelte eine gute compliance gegenüber den Supplementen wieder. Dagegen lässt die sehr hohe Prävalenz an Eisenmangel trotz bereitgestellter Eisensulfat-Tabletten eine niedrige Akzeptanz gegenüber den Eisen-supplementen bei zugleich unzureichender Nahrungsquellen für Eisen vermuten. Eine verbesserte compliance zu den Eisensupplementen wäre sehr wünschenswert. MAM zeigte einen nachhaltig positiven Effekt auf den Zink- und Eisenstatus bei schwangeren wie auch bei stillenden Frauen. Zusätzliche Zinksupplemente und die Anreicherung von Spurenelementen in bereits sehr gut akzeptierten Nahrungsmitteln wie der Fischpaste wären weitere erfolgversprechende Maßnahmen um die hohe Rate an Eisen- und Zinkmangel zu reduzieren. Vitamin A Mangel scheint kein ernstes Gesundheitsproblem und Serum Retinol war nicht mehr offensichtlich durch DDT Rückstände beeinflusst.

α-Tocopherol, β-Carotene and Thiamin waren positive wohingegen ein hoher Eisenstatus, höchste Hämatokritwerte, erhöhtes AGP und DDT Rückstände in der Schwangerschaft waren negative Prädikatoren für Gewicht und Größenparameter der Neugeborenen. Eisenstatus und Mikronährstoffe könnten einen direkten Einfluss auf das fötale Wachstum ausüben oder sind Parameter für andere Faktoren die für eine gesunde und erfolgreiche Schwangerschaft verantwortlich sein könnten. Hoher Eisenstatus, hohes Serum Retinol und höchste Hematokritwerte, vor allem im 3. Trimester, scheinen eine unzureichende Blutverdünnung mit daraus folgendem reduziertem Blutfluss über die Plazenta und somit Hemmung der fötalen Entwicklung wiederzuspiegeln. Höheres α-Tocopherol könnte ganz einfach die Konsequenz des vermehrten Konsums von Pflanzenöl sein oder aber einen positiv ausgeglichenen Antioxidantienstatus reflektieren.

Der Einfluss von Thiamin auf das in utero Längenwachstum ist eine bemerkenswerte Beobachtung, welche die Supplementierung mit Thiamin als eine höchst effiziente Maßnahme zur Verbesserung der Neugeborenengröße in einer Gesellschaft, in der jede dritte Schwangere < 150 cm groß ist, demonstriert. Der negative Einfluss von DDT in utero auf das Geburtsgewicht war trotz statistischer Signifikanz verhältnismäßig gering. Deutlichere Effekte auf Schwangerschaftsverlauf, foetales Wachstum und Mikronährstoffe könnten sich in anderen endemischen Malaria-gebieten zeigen, in denen DDT noch aktuell eingesetzt wird. Allerdings sollten hier für eine umfassende Bewertung der Vorteil des DDTs als das bis heute effektivste Insektizid zur Kontrolle der Malaria sowie die Folgen und Risiken in der Schwanger-schaft an Malaria zu erkranken als Argumente für den DDT Einsatz berücksichtigt werden.

Abbreviations

AGP	α-1 Glycoprotein
ANC	Antenatal Care
AOR	Adjusted Odds Ratio
Adj.R^2	Adjusted Variance
BMI	Body Mass Index
BW	Birth Weight
CI	Confidence Interval (usually given as 95% CI)
CRP	C-Reactive Protein
DDE	Dichloro-Diphenyl-Dichloroethylene
DDT	Dichloro-Diphenyl-Trichloroethane
DVM	Delayed Visual Maturation Type I Syndrome
EGA	Estimated Gestational Age
Hb	Hemoglobin
Hct	Hematocrit
IUGR	Intra-Uterine Growth Retardation (LBW at term)
LBW	Low Birth Weight (< 2,500g)
MEF	Micronutrient Enriched Flour
MSF	Médecins Sans Frontières
OR	Odds Ratio
PP	Post Partum
PW	Pregnant Women
PF	*Plasmodium falciparum* malaria
PV	*Plasmodium vivax* malaria
SF	Serum ferritin
SMRU	Shoklo Malaria Research Unit
sTfR	soluble Transferrin Receptor
TBBC	Thai-Burma Border Consortium
TDP	Thiamine Di-Phosphate
TMP	Thiamine Mono-Phosphate
VAD	Vitamin A Deficiency
WHO	World Health Organization

1. Introduction

1.1 Ante-natal care (ANC) by the SMRU in Maela camp

Since 1984, thousands of displaced people from neighbouring Myanmar, mainly of Karen ethnic origin, have taken refuge in Thailand. In 2006, their number exceeded 150,000. Refugee camps are located in four different provinces bordering Myanmar. Maela camp, located in Mae Ramat district, Tak province, Northern Thailand (**Fig. 1**: K3) is the largest settlement with up to 50,000 inhabitants (CCSDTP, TBBC, 2006).

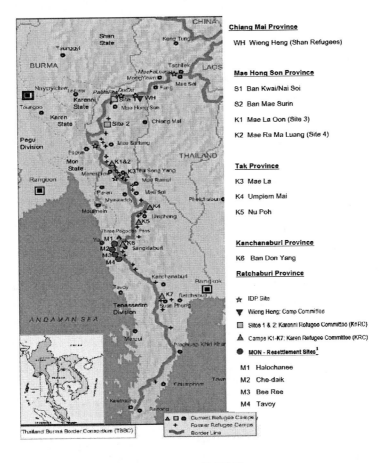

Chiang Mai Province

WH Wieng Heng (Shan Refugees)

Mae Hong Son Province

S1 Ban Kwai/Nai Soi

S2 Ban Mae Surin

K1 Mae La Oon (Site 3)

K2 Mae Ra Ma Luang (Site 4)

Tak Province

K3 Mae La

K4 Umpiem Mai

K5 Nu Poh

Kanchanaburi Province

K6 Ban Don Yang

Ratchaburi Province

★   IDP Site

▼   Wieng Heng: Camp Committee

▨   Sites 1 & 2: Karonni Refugee Committee (KnRC)

▲   Camps K1-K7: Karen Refugee Committee (KRC)

●   MON - Resettlement Sites[1]

M1 Halochanee

M2 Che-daik

M3 Bee Ree

M4 Tavoy

▲ ▨ ● Current Refugee Camps
+ Former Refugee Camps
Border Line

Fig.1 Border Map December 2006 (curtesy of TBBC)

Established in 1986, the Shoklo Malaria Research Unit (SMRU) (www.shoklo-unit.com) is a field station attached to the Hospital for Tropical Diseases, Mahidol University, Bangkok, and is part of the Mahidol-Oxford University Research Unit (http://www.tropmedres.ac/). The unit primarily provides malaria diagnostic and treatment services to populations living in the camps for displaced people in this area of extreme multi-drug resistant falciparum malaria. In 1985, the malaria related maternal mortality rate was very high with an estimated 10 deaths per 1,000 live births (Nosten, 1991). Since 1986, the SMRU has been providing antenatal and delivery services to the Karen ethnic minority living in the camps. A system of weekly antenatal care (ANC) has been developed where women have regular checks on malaria risk, hematocrit levels, blood pressure measurements, fundal height measurements, weight, and estimation of gestational age by ultrasound. They have the opportunity to receive tetanus vaccinations and treatment for inter-current medical and obstetrical problems and have the possibility to deliver in the unit. Almost 90% of the pregnant women in the camps follow the weekly ANC consultation. Malaria, still one of the most common morbid events, has been drastically reduced in the 1990s; with the last maternal death attributed to malaria in 1994 (Nosten 2000). Beside malaria and other infectious diseases, deficiency of iron and micronutrients remains one of the major health problems in Maela camp.

1.2 Iron, thiamine and micronutrient deficiencies

Iron and micronutrient deficiencies affect people in nearly all developing countries and are highly prevalent in long-term refugees and internally displaced populations (Toole 1992, Prinzo 2002, Woodruff 2006). During pregnancy, as a period of increased metabolic demand, inadequate stores or intake of vitamins and minerals can affect maternal health, pregnancy outcomes and infant development (Ramakrishnan 1999, Allen 2005).

In the late 1980s, thiamine deficiency was recognized as the main cause (40%) of the extremely high infantile mortality (18%) in Maela camp; early diagnosis and prompt treatment of severe vitamin B1 deficiency in infants decreased mortality attributable to beri-beri from 73 to 5 per 1000 live birth (Luxemburger 2003).

Iron and micronutrient malnutrition remains prevalent as nutrition relies mainly on the provided food basket which is adequate in energy and protein, but low in iron and micronutrients such as vitamin A, folate and thiamine (Riedel 1997, Banjong 2003). Deficiency of thiamine and vitamin A as well as high prevalence of anemia has been documented in pregnant and postpartum women in this population (Luxemburger 2001, McGready 2001, Stuetz 2006). Further a delay in visual maturation (DVM) was found in over 90% of a cohort of newborns from Maela camp (McGready 2003). This neurological syndrome, for the first time described in a population, is most likely explained by a micronutrient deficiency or a combination of micronutrients deficit, and maybe aggravated by the toxic effects of residual DDT.

1.3 DDT exposure and common habits of women in the camps

Over the span of 50 years, Dichloro-Diphenyl-Trichloroethane (DDT) has been used as an insecticide for malaria control in Northern Thailand. Malaria rates have been dramatically decreased in Thailand as a result of successful vector control based primarily on the use of DDT for residual house spraying (Chareonviriyaphap 2000). International pressure and perceived adverse impact on environment and human health contributed to the decision to replace DDT by synthetic pyrethroids (phase out period 1995-1999). In Maela camp DDT indoor-residual spraying took place between 1995 and 2000, and was then replaced by the pyrethroid Deltamethrin. However, high serum DDT residues which affected serum retinol levels were detected among pregnant women living in Maela camp (Stuetz 2006). DDT may additionally affect thiamine status; long-term administration of DDT in rats resulted in thiamine deficiency despite its sufficient dietary intake (Yagi 1979). The possible implication by DDT in reproductive health and infant development is still under debate. Some studies have described an association between DDT or its metabolite DDE and an increased risk of abortion (Korrik 2001), preterm delivery and small-for gestational age babies (Longnecker 2001); other studies have failed to find any significant association (Farhang 2005, Khanjani 2006, Fenster 2006).

A high proportion (approximately 30%) of pregnant women from the camps smoke cheroots, cigars 15 cm in length and constist of a white dried betel nut leaf wrapper filled with coarse ground tobacco (McGready et al 1998). In this population smoking during pregnancy was associated with a 1.8 fold increased risk of low birth weight and a mean birth weight reduction of 159 g (95%CI 83-235 g) compared to non-smokers, after adjusting for confounders. Although they smoke on average only 1-2 cheroots per day the intake of carbon monoxide and nicotine as analysed in the UK at the Laboratory of the Government Chemist using internationally approved standards was estimated to be similar to European women who smoke about 10 or more cigarettes each day.

An even higher proportion (≥80%) of pregnant women consumes betel nut (McGready 2001, Luxemburger 2003). Betel quid chewing is an ancient practice common in many Asian countries (Gupta 2004). The basic quid is made from the betel leaf (Piper betel), with the chopped or crushed nut from the areca palm (seed of the fruit *Areca catechu L.* palm tree, which grows or is cultivated in almost every part of Thailand and Burma), and a white (or pink) paste of slaked lime (calcium hydroxide). The pharmacological and adverse effects of betel quid chewing are caused by the alkaloids and tannins released from the areca nut. The mature green betel leaves contain volatile oils, nitrates and small quantities of sugar, startch and tannins. In Northern Thailand, both smoking habits and and betel nut chewing was associated with oral cancer (Reichart 1990). Betel quid chewing during pregnancy was associated with an increased risk of adverse birth outcomes among aborigines in Taiwan (Yang 1999, 2001). Regularly consumption of betel nut and raw fish presents a real problem in populations whose diets are borderline thiamine sufficient as the betel nut and raw fish contains antithiamine factors (Vimokesant 1975, Davis 1983).

1.4 Provision of food rations, supplements, and micronutrient enriched flour

All adults in the Thai-Burmese border refugee camps received a general monthly food ration including 16 kg of rice, 1.5 kg of split mung beans, 1 kg of fermented fish, 300 g iodized salt, 914 grams (1litre) soybean oil and 125 g dried chillies (**Table 1.1**). In July 2004 micronutrient enriched whole wheat flour with basic vitamins and minerals were introduced to all inhabitants of Maela camp. This additional food ration to improve the supply of micronutrients could play an important role for pregnant and breast-feeding women. Each adult was provided with 1.4 kg of MEF per month and the rations of rice and of mung bean were reduced to 15 and 1 kg respectively. Later in March 2005 whole wheat flour was replaced by the rice flour based 'Asia Mix' (**Table 1.3**).

14

Since 1997, additional supplementary food ration provided by TBBC and delivered by SMRU has been provided to women attending the antenatal care consultations in the clinics. The weekly supplementary ration includes 500 grams split mung beans and 300 grams (200 g for lactating women) dried fish. In February 2005 red beans and tinned fish instead of split mung beans and dried fish, respectively, and additional 250 ml vegetable oil were provided (**Table 1.1**).

Table 1.1 General food baskets for adults and additional food rations for pregnant and breast feeding women during ANC consultation

Food basket per month	until 30 June 2004	1 July 2004 on going
Fortified flour **(MEF)**	0 kg	**1.4 kg**
Rice	16 kg	15 kg
Split mung bean	1,5 kg	1 kg
Fermented fish / sea fish	1 kg	1 kg / 750 g [a]
Iodized salt	300 g	300 g
Soybean oil	914 g (1litre)	914 g (1 litre)
Dried chillies	125 g	125 g
Additional food per week	**March 2004 - Feb 2005**	**Feb 2005 on going**
Split mung bean	500 g	
Red beans		500 g
Dried fish	300 g	
Tinned fish		310 g (2 tins)
Vegetable oil		230 g (250 ml)

[a] in March 2005 fermented fish was replaced by 750 gram cleaned sea fish.

SMRU has provided vitamin supplements to pregnant women since it's inception in 1986. Since 1998 and during the study period micronutrient supplements for pregnant women consisted of thiamine (7 x 100mg thiamine mononitrate-B1 NO_3), folate (7 x 5 mg folic acid) and iron (7x 600mg iron sulphate -$FeSO_4$) and were provided weekly during ANC consultations (**Table 1.2**). At delivery all women receive systematically 200,000 IU (208 µmol) of vitamin A in the form of retinyl palmitate. Post partum mothers were still weekly provided with thiamine supplements (7 x 100mg) and the additional food rations as during pregnancy.

Table 1.2 Provided micronutrient- and iron supplements during pregnancy

Weekly provided supplements for pregnant women during ANC consultation	
Thiamine	7 x 100 mg thiamine mono-nitrate ≈ 7 x 93 mg thiamine chloride
Folate	7 x 5 mg folic acid
Iron	7 x 600 mg ferrous sulphate ≈ 7x 200 mg elemental iron

Table 1.3 Composition of micronutrient enriched flour (per 100 gram), based on the recommendation by World Food Programme / Codex Alimentarius

		Whole wheat flour	Asia mix
Whole wheat / Refined rice flour		75% whole wheat	75% rice flour
Soy bean flour (precooked)		25%	25%
kcal per 100 grams [kcal]		415	400
Protein (per 100 gr)		14.5 g (14.5%)	14 g (14%)
Fat (per 100 gr)		2.8 g (2.8%)	6 g (6%)
Micronutrients	**Fortification / 100g**	**Final concentration per 100 grams**	
Vitamin A (RE)*	500 / 500 (600) RE	500 RE	500 RE (600)
Thiamine (NO_3)	0.18 / 0.9 (1.0) mg	0.6 mg	0.9 mg (1.0)
Riboflavin (univer)	0.45 / 1.5 (2.5) mg	0.6 mg	1.5 mg (2.5)
Niacin (amide)	4.8 / 4.8 (5.6) mg	7.6 mg	4.8 mg (5.6)
Folate (folic acid)	60 (120) / 160 µg	60 µg	160 µg
Vit C (ascorb. acid)	48 / 48 mg	48 mg	48 mg
Vit B12 (0.1%WS)	1.2 / 1.2 (1.4) µg	1.2 µg	1.2 µg (1.4)
Zinc (sulphate)	5 / 5 (10) mg	8 mg	5 mg (10)
Iron (fumarate)	8 (16) / 20 mg	19 mg	24.5 mg
Calcium (CO_3)	100 / 100 mg	196 mg	192.5 mg

* RE: retinol equivalent (500 RE = 500 µg retinol ≈ 1664 IU)

1.5 Objectives of the study

In June-July 2004 a cross-sectional study among pregnant (1st to 3rd trimester) and post partum women (12 weeks pp, n=89) was conducted to assess micronutrient status and DDT exposure prior to the introduction of the enriched flour. All these pregnant women were followed up at weekly ANC until delivery and 100 mother-infant pairs, provided for the first time with fortified flour were followed as a cohort until 3 months post-partum. A second cross-sectional study among pregnant women was conducted in November 2006, more than 2 years after the introduction of the enriched flour; women were followed for blood- and breast-milk samples at 3 months post partum. The overall aim of the cross-sectional and cohort studies was to characterize status and changes in iron, thiamine and micronutrients as well as exposure to DDT during pregnancy and in the post partum period. The specific objectives were to

- Assess the impact by provided iron and micronutrient supplements and introduced micronutrient enriched flour in Maela camp
- Identify predictors for iron and micronutrient deficiencies
- Determine residues and predictors of DDT exposure
- Analyse the impact by micronutrients and DDT exposure on newborn weight, length and arm- and head circumference

2. Methods

2.1 Study design and recruitment

Between 2004 and 2008, two cross-sectional surveys with subsequent follow-up studies as shown in the flow chart **Fig. 2.1a, b** were conducted in the ante-natal care clinics of the SMRU in Maela camp, 50 km north of Mae Sot at the Thai Myanmar Border. All pregnant women independently of their gestational age and lactating women in week 12 post partum attending the ANC consultation were eligible for participation. The project was approved by the Faculty of Tropical Medicine of Mahidol University, and the Oxford Tropical Research Ethics Committee, University of Oxford. Recruitment was organised as cross-sectional studies in June 2004 and November 2006. The purpose and the methods of the survey were explained to all participants in their own language and they were free to withdraw from the study at any time and without consequences. Exclusion criteria included not receiving the regular monthly food ration from the camp (not registered), living outside the camp, a hematocrit < 20% recorded the week before or the day of the survey, and/or hospitalization in the In-Patient Department (IPD) on the day of the survey. Pregnant women who intended to deliver outside Maela camp or to leave the camp immediately after delivery were also excluded.

Group 1: pregnant women - **PW 1** (n=534)	**Group PP:** post partum women - **PP** (n=89)
• questionnaires, clinical examinations • blood sample to analyse MNs and DDT • ANC, pregnancy outcomes	• SMRU-ANC, pregnancy outcomes • blood and milk sample to analyse MNs and DDT

Introduction of enriched flour in the camp, July 2004

Follow-up

(Sept-Nov 06)

Group 1: mothers post partum - **PP1 (PPEF[**])** (n=100)
• blood and milk sample at week 12 post partum for the analysis on MNs and DDT

Fig. 2.1a Cross-sectional survey among pregnant (PW1) and post partum women (PP) in June 2004, and follow-up of 100 mothers in post partum (PP1)

[**] PPEF: post partum women who received the micronutrient enriched whole wheat flour

```
┌─────────────────────────────────────────────────────────────────────┐
│           Group 2: pregnant women - PW 2 (n=515)                      │
│   •   questionnaires, clinical examinations                           │
│   •   blood sample to analyse MNs and DDT residues                    │
│   •   ANC, pregnancy outcome (birth weight, infants anthropometry)    │
└─────────────────────────────────────────────────────────────────────┘
```

follow-up in week 12 pp   February - August 2007

```
┌─────────────────────────────────────────────────────────────────────┐
│           Group 2: mothers post partum - PP 2 (n=485)                 │
│   •   blood and milk sample to analyse MNs and DDT residues           │
└─────────────────────────────────────────────────────────────────────┘
```

Fig. 2.1b Second cross-sectional survey among pregnant women in November 2006 (PW2), and follow-up in post partum (PP2)

2.2 Baseline characteristics, clinical examinations and antenatal care (ANC)

Provided that written informed consent was obtained, questionnaires, clinical examination and sampling of blood specimens were performed the week of enrolment. A structured interview questionnaire was used to collect information on maternal socio-demographic, medical, reproductive, and life style characteristics. Baseline demographic data of the women such as age, height, weight, gravidity, and parity as well as hematocrit measurements were generally registered at entry to prenatal care. After enrolment, pregnant women continued to follow the routine weekly ANC until delivery.

Hematocrit values <30% were regarded as low levels indicating anemia. Gestational age was estimated by ultrasound measurements at first consultation (between 8-12 weeks) and again around 18 weeks (17 to 22 weeks). So in general, women had one or 2 ultrasounds during their pregnancy. If a woman had her first ultrasound after 22nd week of pregnancy, then the gestational age at delivery was confirmed by doing the Dubowitz test (Dubowitz, 1977). The best estimate of gestational age was used for each woman and priority was given to early ultrasound scan, 18 week ultrasound scan, or Dubowitz if the first ultrasound was very late (>24 weeks).

Body mass index (kg/m^2) was calculated from the weight and height taken at admission. In addition, for 23% of the women (266/1137) who didn't come for a first trimester ANC consultation (EGA ≥ week 13) weight was individually back corrected to gestational week 9 (EGA 9) using following regression:

Weight EGA 9 = weight ≥ week 13 - (weight for EGA ≥ week 13 - weight for EGA 9),

whereby estimated weight for gestational age (weight for EGA) ≥ week 13 and at week 9 (weight for EGA 9) were calculated by following equation based on the median of weights taken in trimester 1 (47.0 kg at EGA 8.3 weeks, n=889), trimester 2 and of serial weight measurements in week 18, 24, 28, 32, and 36:

Weight for EGA [kg] = -0.0004 EGA^2 + 0.304 EGA + 44.65 kg   (R^2=0.987).

Normal values of BMI for the Asian population as proposed by the WHO range between 18.5 to 23.0 kg/m^2 (WHO Expert Consultation, 2004); values < 18.5 kg/m^2 and ≥ 23 kg/m^2 were used as cut-offs indicating underweight and overweight (obesity) in women with first trimester data.

2.3 Pregnancy outcomes measures

Primary outcomes were birth weight and gestational duration. Newborn birth weight and placenta weight were measured with an electronic scale (Seca 335, Hamburg, Germany, precision 10 gram). Weights of singleton births were assessed whereas abortions, stillbirths with less than 1000 gram (1 case in PW1), twins and newborn weights measured at or later than day 4 (>72 hours after delivery) were excluded from statistical analysis. Birth weights taken on day 2 and day 3 were corrected for the fact of weight loss by 3.6% (95% CI: -3.9 to -3.4%) and 4.4% (95% CI: -4.7 to -4.1%) respectively. The weight loss of 3.6% until day 2 and 4.4% until day 3 are mean values from a follow-up study among 380 infants (54% male) born in Maela camp in 2007 (unpublished data, Claudia Turner and Verena Carrara). Corrected birth weights were computed as follows:

Birth weight day 1 [grams] = Birth weight day 2 * (1/ (1-(3.642/100)))
= Birth weight day 3 * (1/ (1-(4.365/100)))

Abortion was defined as pregnancy ending before 28 weeks gestation while a stillbirth was defined as a delivery with a dead newborn (foetal death) from 28 weeks of gestation (≥ 28.0 wks). Low birth weight (LBW) was defined as any newborn weighing less than 2500 g, independent of the gestational age, prematurity as a delivery before 37 weeks' gestation (<37.0 wks), and intra-uterine growth retardation (IUGR) as a newborn with LBW born at term (birth weight < 2500 g and EGA at outcome ≥ 37 weeks). Newborns were considered small for gestational age (SGA) if birth weight was at or below the 10th percentile at each week of gestation, with the 'valid' birth weights in the weeks 34-42 of the present study as a standard (**Table 2.1**).

Table 2.1 Small for gestational age (SGA): birth weight ≤10th percentile of birth weight at each week of gestation

EGA at birth * [weeks]	N	Birth weight (BW) ** [grams]	Percentile 10 [grams]	N ≤10th Centile
34	10	2142 (241)	1800	2
35	19	2457 (318)	2100	2
36	30	2593 (286)	2200	4
37	101	2815 (348)	2392	10
38	230	2900 (412)	2362	23
39	356	3018 (377)	2530	36
40	221	3197 (377)	2714	22
41	90	3324 (440)	2771	9
42	9	3279 (416)	2530	1

*EGA at birth: estimated gestational age at birth outcome; ** BW in mean (SD)

Secondary outcome variables included newborn length, arm circumference and head circumference. Newborn length was assessed on a measuring mat (Seca 210, Hamburg, Germany, precision 1cm) while head and arm circumference were assessed with a measuring tape (Seca 202, Hamburg, Germany, precision 1 mm).

2.4 Sample collection

Capillary blood was taken for hematocrit measurements done in the SMRU antenatal clinics. Non-fasting blood samples including EDTA-whole blood and whole blood for serum were collected between 10.00 and 12.00 am by venepuncture into vacutainers that were wrapped in aluminium foil. Breast-milk samples were collected by manual expression into glass tubes (Pyrex), again wrapped in aluminium foil in order to protect against degradation of photosensitive substances (vitamin E, carotenoids) by direct sunlight. Whole blood, serum and breast-milk were portioned into Eppendorf tubes, then subsequently frozen at -20°C in Maela camp before being transported to the SMRU office in Mae Sot to be stored at -80°C.

Frozen samples were sent on dry ice to Chiang Mai (Research Institute for Health Sciences) for the analysis on DDT residues and to the University of Hohenheim, Stuttgart (Institute of Biological Chemistry and Nutrition) for the analysis on vitamins, zinc, copper cholesterol and triglycerides. Finally aliquots of serum were transferred to DBS-Tech, Willstaett (Dr. JG Erhardt) for the determination on serum ferritin (SF), soluble transferrin receptor (sTfR) and the acute phase proteins CRP and AGP. Sample size varied slightly across the DDT and micronutrient determinations because of insufficient quantities of specimens in individual cases.

2.5 Laboratory analysis: micronutrients and DDT residues in blood and milk

2.5.1 Fat soluble vitamins (retinol, tocopherol, carotenoids) in serum and breast-milk

Extraction and HPLC analysis of serum retinol, α-tocopherol, and β-carotene were performed as previously described (Stuetz, 2006). Certified NIST standards (Gaithersburg, MD, USA) were used for quantification. Pooled serum analysed within each batch (n=12) of samples gave inter-batch CVs for serum retinol (5.3%), α-tocopherol (5.6%) and β-carotene (5.7%) of < 6%.

Fat soluble vitamins retinol, tocopherols and carotenoids in milk were analysed as follows: to each 10 ml screw top glass tube containing 0.5 ml of thawed milk sample and a magnet for stirring, 1 ml ethanol containing β-apo-8'-carotenal-methyloxime as internal standard (Sommerburg, 1997) and 2.5% (wt/vol) pyrogallol was added followed by 0.5 ml 50% (wt/vol) KOH solution. Tubes were closed with screw caps and kept in a covered water bath (Ramazotti) at 38°C, being placed on a stirrer, for saponification under constant stirring. After 2 hours 2 ml of 15% NaCl-solution was added and vitamins were extracted twice with 1 ml of hexane. Combined hexane layers were washed with 7.5% NaCl-solution and transferred to tubes for evaporation under nitrogen. Residues were re-dissolved in ethanol and mobile phase (1:3) in order to be analysed on a Varian-HPLC (Pro Star 210) with same chromatographic conditions as for serum vitamins: ODS-2 analytical column (3 µm, 250 x 4.6 mm, Trentec, Gerlingen) at 40°C and a mobile phase consisting acetonitril, dioxin, and methanol (82:15:3) in recirculation mode with a flow rate of 1.5 ml/min. Retinol and carotenoids were detected at 325 and 450 nm while α-tocopherol was measured by fluorescence (excitation/emission set at 298/328 nm). For calibration three different serum pools with assigned values set against Standard Reference Material (SRM 968c, NIST, Gaithersburg, MD) were treated as described above for milk samples. Vitamin levels were confirmed by a standard mixture (Standards from running on each day of analysis. Pooled milk was analysed within each batch of samples (n=12) giving inter-assay CVs for retinol (5.4%), lutein/zeaxanthin (8.3%), β-cryptoxanthin (6.6%), α-tocopherol (6.6%) and β-carotene (7.9%) of < 9%.

Serum retinol < 0.7 µmol/L and < 1.05 µmol/L were used as cut-offs indicating vitamin A deficiency (VAD) and low vitamin A status, respectively. Breast milk retinol ≤ 1.05 µmol/L milk and ≤ 8 µg/g milk fat (28 µmol/kg milk fat) were considered indicative of low breast-milk vitamin A content (WHO, 1996). Serum α-tocopherol < 11.6 µmol/L and α-tocopherol-cholesterol ratio < 2.2 µmol/L/mmol/L were regarded as deficient vitamin E status (Sauberlich 1999, Thurnham 1986).

2.5.2 Cholesterol and triglycerides in serum and fat in human milk

Serum cholesterol and triglycerides were analysed by enzymatic methods using diagnostic kits (ABX, Esslingen and Olympus, Hamburg) adapted for the Cobas Mira and Olympus AT200 auto analyzer. Milk fat was determined as described by Lucas et al (1987); milk aliquots of 50 µl were diluted (1:20) with 950 µl of a Triton/EDTA mixture and placed in a water bath at 60^0C for 15 min to achieve complete clarification before being analysed by the enzymatic method as for serum triglycerides. For quality control pooled serum and milk was analysed along with each batch of samples giving between assay CVs for serum cholesterol, serum triglycerides and milk triglycerides with the Cobas Mira of 2.1%, 7.6% and 4.8%, and with the Olympus AT200 of 3.2%, 5.2% and 6.8%, respectively.

2.5.3 Thiamine in whole blood and breast-milk

Thiamine and its phosphate esters in whole blood and breast milk samples were determined using precolumn derivatization, reversed-phase liquid chromatography and fluorescence detection as described by Gerrits et al (1997) with modification. In brief 500 µl of EDTA- whole blood or human milk was deproteinized by the addition of cold perchloric acid (7%PCA); 500 µl of supernatant was derivatised with 100 µl freshly prepared thiochromation reagent (12 mM $K_3Fe(CN)_6$ in 3.35 M NaOH). Finally pH was adjusted to 7 by addition of 20µl of 5M phosphoric acid (to stop reaction) and 20 µl were analysed on a Merck Hitachi HPLC (LaChrom) equipped with autosampler (L-7250), colomn oven (L-7360; set at 40^0C), solvent degaser (L-7612) and fluorescence detector (L-7480; excitation/emission set at 367/435 nm). The separation of thiamine di-phosphate (TDP) in whole blood and thiamine monophophate (TMP) and thiamine in human milk was achieved using a 5 µm analytical column (Grom-Sil, 120 ODS-4 HE, 125 x 4 mm, Grom, Germany) and a mobile phase consisting methanol (17.5% V/V for whole blood and 27,5% V/V for milk) and phosphate buffer (pH 7) at a flow rate of 0.8 ml/min. Data were acquired, processed and evaluated with the Clarity chromatographic station, DA-C50 (DataApex Ltd, Praha). The limit of detection of the method (LDM: 10 x noise) for thiamine and its phosphate esters was ≤ 2 µg/L.

External calibration curves from TDP (Sigma Chemicals), TMP and thiamine hydrochloride standards (Fluka, 95160) prepared by serial dilution into 0.1 M HCl were used for quantification. For internal quality control pools of whole blood and milk were analysed within each batch (n=12) of samples giving inter-batch CV's for whole blood TDP of 6.6% (<7%) and for TMP (4.2%) and thiamine (3.5%) in milk of < 5%. Whole blood TDP <30 µg/L (65 nmol/L) adapted to low whole blood TDP levels in Japanese volunteers (Ihara, 2005) and lowest whole blood total thiamine and TDP (70nM) in Europe (Wielders, 1983, Schrijver, 1982, Floridi, 1984) was considered as a cut off value for low thiamine status. Breast milk thiamine <100 µg/L was considered indicative of low levels and deficiency of thiamine (WHO, 1999).

2.5.4 Indicators for iron status (SF, sTfR), infection markers and iron in milk

Serum ferritin (SF), soluble transferring receptor (sTfR), C-reactive protein (CRP), and α-1 glycoprotein (AGP) were measured by ELISA using polyclonal (DAKO, Finland: SF, CRP, AGP) and monoclonal antibodies (Hytest, Finland: sTfR). Serum quality material (Liquicheck, BIORAD) was used for quantification and all assays were done in duplicate. Serum pools measured as a quality control (n=8 per plate) gave between-assay coefficients of variations of 2.9%, 4%, 2.5% and 3% for SF, sTfR, CRP, and AGP, respectively. The assays had a sensitivity of 2 μg/L for SF, 0.5 mg/L for sTfR, 0.1 mg/L for CRP and 0.05 g/L for AGP.

Total body iron stores were calculated using SF and sTfR in an equation proposed by Cook et al. (2003): body iron (mg/kg) = - [$\log_{10}$ (sTfR x 1000/SF) - 2.8229] / 0.1207. Positive values represent storage iron while negative values indicate a deficit in tissue iron in subjects with iron deficiency.

Iron deficiency was defined by serum ferritin (SF) <12 μg/L (Skikne, 1990, Cook, 1992) or sTfR >8.5 mg/L (Skikne, 1990). Anemia was defined as Hb< 110 g/L for pregnant women in 1st and 2nd trimester, as Hb< 105 g/L for pregnant women in trimester 2 and as Hb <120 g/l for those women in post partum (CDC, 1989, WHO, 2001). Iron deficiency anemia (IDA) was defined by the simultaneous presence of iron deficiency and anemia (Cook JD, 2005, Berger 2005). CRP >10 μg/L and AGP >1g/L were used as cut-offs defining an acute phase response by infection or inflammation (Semba 2000).

Iron in breast milk was analysed by Inductively Coupled Plasma Optical Emission Spectrometry (ICP-OES) after microwave-assisted digestion. Samples of 1 ml were mineralized with (2 ml) concentrated nitric acid (65% HNO_3) for 2 hours in a closed-pressurized, high performance microwave digestion unit (MLS Ultra Clave, MLS GmbH, Leutkirch). Completely clear homogenous digests were diluted to 10 ml with high-purity water in order to be analysed by ICP-OES on a Varian Vista Pro Radial.

2.5.5 Zinc and copper in serum and breast milk

Zinc and copper in serum were analysed by inductively coupled plasma mass spectrometry (ICP-MS). In falcon tubes, 100 μl of internal standard solution (1mg/L, Rhodium (III) chloride, Merck, Darmstadt) was added to 100 μl serum and filled up to 10 ml with de-ionized water (1:50 dilution) in order to be analysed by ICP-MS on an Elan 6000, Perkin Elmer Sciex. Calibration with ICP multi-element standard solution VI (CertiPur, Merck, Darmstadt) was done on each day of analysis. Human control sera (Seronorm Trace Elements, SERO AS, Norway) measured agreed well with the certified values. For internal quality control pooled serum was analysed within each batch (n=20) of samples giving inter-batch CV's for zinc and copper of 5.3 and 4.1%, respectively. Serum zinc deficient values were defined using the following suggested cut-offs for pregnant and non-pregnant women: 0.56 mg/L for trimester 1, 0.50 mg/L for trimester 2 and 3 and 0.66 mg/L for non-pregnant women (Hotz, 2003).

Zinc and copper in milk were analysed as described by Nobrega et al. (1997) with modification. 500 µl of milk together with 0.1 ml internal standard solution (Rhodium (III) chloride, 1 mg/L) was dissolved in 9.4 ml (was filled up to 10 ml with) 5% v/v mixed tertiary amines-EDTA reagent at pH 8 (CFA-C Reagent, Spectrasol, Warwick, NY) before being analysed by ICP-MS as described for serum samples. Pooled milk (n=25) analysed along 184 specimens gave CV's of 3.6% for zinc and of 5.2% for copper.

2.5.6 DDT and its metabolites (DDE, DDD) in serum and breast milk

DDT (p,p'-DDT) and its metabolites were determined in 2 ml of serum or breast milk according to a method by Prapamontol and Stevenson (1991) with modifications described previously (Stuetz, 2001, 2006). In brief, after extraction and clean-up using solid-phase extraction, compounds were eluted with isooctane and analysed on a Hewlett-Packard 5890 A series II gas chromatograph equipped with an automatic sampler (HP 7673), a fused silica capillary column (Ultra 2: 25 m x 0.32 mm i.d., with 0.52 µm film thickness), and a ^{63}Ni electron-capture detector. Spiked bovine serum and cow milk were used for calibration. Mean recoveries of spiked bovine serum ranged from 98% for p,p'-DDT to 103% for p,p'-DDD. Recoveries in spiked cow milk ranged from 97% for p,p'-DDD to 105% for p,p'-DDE and p,p'-DDT. The detection limit of the method (signal to noise ratio of 10:1) ranged from 0.04 ng/ml for p,p'-DDE to 0.1 ng/ml for p,p'-DDT. Results were not corrected for recoveries and values less than the LDM of 0.1 ng/ml were regarded as zero and not detected. For internal quality control one sample of pooled human serum or human milk was analysed along with each batch (n=8) of specimens giving inter-batch CVs of 4.2%, 8.5%, and 4.4% for p,p'-DDE, p,p'-DDT and total DDT (sum of p,p'-DDE, p,p'-DDD, o,p'-DDT, and p,p'-DDT), respectively. The precision and accuracy of the method were assessed through participation in the External Intercomparison Programme 36 (in 2005) and 40 (in 2007) of the German External Quality Assessment Scheme (G-EQUAS 36 and 40).

Determined values for DDE and DDT in high (2 levels in occupational-medical range) and low (2 levels in environmental-medical range) concentrations agreed well with the certified values (within the tolerance range ± 3s of reference values).

DDT levels are also expressed on the lipid weight basis. Therefore total lipids in serum were estimated by the following regression using serum concentrations of triglycerides and cholesterol as proposed by Rylander et al., 2005:

Total lipids [g/L] = 0.92 + 1.31 *(cholesterol + triglycerides).

2.6 Data analysis, statistics

All statistical analyses were conducted with SPSS for WINDOWS (SPSS Inc., Chicago, IL; Version 11.5); two-tailed P values < 0.05 were considered statistically significant. Continuous normal distributed variables were described by their mean (SD, range) and non-normally distributed variables by their median (range) or geometric mean (2SD range, +/- 1SD). Percentages were given for categorical and binary data. Means between groups were compared by Student's t-test and one-way ANOVA post-hoc tests (Scheffe, Dunnett). Data that were not normally distributed were transformed using log or square root transformations, as appropriate. In addition, significant differences between skewed data were confirmed by the non-parametric tests (Mann-Whitney U, Kruskal-Wallis H and Wilcoxon test). Bivariate associations were assessed by Pearson's product moment and Spearman's rank correlation. Chi-square tests and logistic regression were applied to compare prevalence and proportions of categorical variables between groups while linear regression analysis was used to assess predictors for continuous outcome variables.

For the comparison of micronutrients, DDT levels and pregnancy outcomes women were separated into 3 main groups: a separate post partum women group (PP), a first pregnant women group (PW1) and a second group of pregnant women (PW2). PP and PW1 were women from the first (2004) while PW2 represents women from the second cross-sectional study (2006). Women of PW1 and PW2 were separated into trimester of pregnancy (T1, T2, T3) when blood samples were taken, and in both groups women were followed (20% of PW1, and 90% of PW2) after delivery for a blood draw and milk sample in week 12 post partum (PP1 and PP2).

Overall two groups of pregnant women (PW1, PW2) separated into trimesters of pregnancy (T1, T2, T3) and 3 post partum women groups (PP, PP1, PP2) were assessed for status and changes in iron, micronutrients and DDT residues. The mean levels of each variable were assessed visually using box plots and tested for significant trend from first to third trimester using linear regression. Mean levels of each variable from the women in the initial post partum group (PP) were then compared with those women who presented in the first trimester (as an approximation for 'baseline') and with the two 'follow up' post partum groups (PP1, PP2) who both received the micronutrient enriched flour. The differences of micronutrient and DDT levels as well as of pregnancy outcome variables between year of sampling (2004 vs. 2006/7) by means of different cross sectional studies (PW1 vs. PW2 and PP/PP1 vs. PP2) were analysed as part of multivariate regression analysis. Forward linear regressions models were used to identify independent predictors of micronutrient and DDT levels and pregnancy outcomes (birth weight, length, arm- and head circumference). Multiple logistic regressions with a forward stepwise approach (Wald) were used to assess predictors and risk factors for iron and micronutrient deficiencies, preterm delivery and infants low birth weight specifying that only variables with p-value <0.05 should be retained in the model. Each nutrient was initially examined separately as a predictor in univariate analysis. The following covariates were examined: maternal age, height and weight (BMI) at first clinical visit (at admission), parity, smoking status (smoker=1), regular daily betel nut (areca) and fermented fish ('nya-u htee') consumption, years of the living in the camp and in Thailand, women's religion (Christian, Buddhist or Muslim) and weeks of individual supplements provided at the time of blood draw. The fit of each linear regression model was controlled by inspecting the residuals. Appropriate model fit of logistic regression was confirmed using the Hosmer-Lemeshow goodness-of-fit test after grouping the data by predicted probabilities of deficiency into ten approximately equal-sized groups.

3. Results

3.1 Maternal socio-demographic and obstetrical characteristics

In June 2004, 764 women were registered in the antanatal clinics of the SMRU in Maela refugee camp. 533 pregnant women (70% - PW1) and 89 breast-feeding mothers (PP) who delivered term singleton babies in March to April gave their written consent and participated to the first cross-sectional study in June to July 2004.

515 out of 745 registered pregnant women (69% - PW2) were recruited for the second cross-sectional survey in November 2006. Maternal characteristics recorded at entry to prenatal care, separated by main groups, are summarized in **Table 3.1.1**. Weight was adjusted to a first trimester weight (weight EGA9) for 23% of the women. The comparison between groups revealed similar age, height, parity and years of staying in Maela or Thailand, whereas weight and BMI in PW2 was significantly higher than in PW1; higher BMI in PW2 is represented by significantly less women with underweight (BMI < 18.5) and more women with over weight than in PW1.

Table 3.1.1 Characteristics of the study population at entry to prenatal care

Characteristics at entry to ANC	Post partum group PP (2004) n=89	Pregnant women PW1 (2004) n=533	Pregnant women PW2 (2006) n=515
EGA [week]	10.0 [4.2 - 36.5]	9.1 [0.6 -32.5]	9.2 [4.5 – 36]
EGA < 13 weeks	69%	76%	78%
Age [years]	25 [15 - 40]	26 [16 - 45]	26 [15 – 48]
Height [cm]	151 [138 - 161]	151 [134 - 168]	151 [130 - 167]
Weight [kg]	48.0 [34 - 80]	48.0 [34 - 81]	48.0 [32 - 90]
Weight EGA9 [kg] [2]	47.0 [34 - 80]	46.5 [31 - 81] [c]	47.3 [31 - 90]
BMI (EGA 9) [kg/m^2] [2]	20.6 [14.9 - 32]	20.3 [15.1 - 33] [b]	20.8 [15.1 - 35.7]
BMI < 18.5 [% (n)] [2]	10 (9)	20 (105) [b]	13 (68)
BMI ≥ 23.0 [% (n)] [2]	13 (12) [d]	17 (89) [d]	21 (109)
Gravidity	3 [1 - 10]	3 [1 - 11]	3 [0 - 14]
Parity [babies born]	2 [0 - 8]	2 [0 - 9]	2 [0 - 11]
Parity 0 [% (n)] [2]	17 (15) [d]	21 (110) [c]	26 (134)
Parity 1 [% (n)] [2]	29 (26) [c]	25 (135) [c]	19 (100)
Parity 2-3 [% (n)]	33 (29)	34 (180)	31 (157)
Parity ≥ 4 [% (n)]	21 (19)	20 (108)	24 (124)

Figures are median [range] and percentages
[2] PW2 different to respective other groups: [a] p<0.001, [b] p<0.01, [c] p<0.05, [d] p<0.1

There were no differences in median gravidity or parity between groups but more nulliparous (parity 0) and less primiparous (parity 1) women in PW2 than in PW1 (p<0.05). Results from the questionnaires at study enrolment are presented in **Table 3.1.2**. Years of staying in Maela camp or in Thailand, proportions of smokers and women who ate daily 2-3 times of fermented fish paste didn't differ between groups. But the frequency of women chewing daily betel nut was significantly higher in PW2 (28%) than in PW1 (20%). The proportion of women or households having their own garden (fruits and vegetables) was in PW2 significantly lower than in PW1 (p=0.014). Significantly more women in PW1 and PP (in 2004) than in PW2 reported to have their own chicken or ducks whereas the proportion of women with own pigs or goats was significantly higher in PW2 (2006) than in PW1 or PP (2004). Only 2 women in PW1 and 3 women in PW2 reported to have a cow. Obviously, between 2004 and the end of 2006, there was a decreasing trend of households with own garden and of families with own chicken or ducks but increasing number of households with either pigs or goats.

Table 3.1.2 Characteristics on life style (at study enrolment)

Characteristics at study enrolment	Post partum PP (2004) n=89	Pregnant women PW1 (2004) n=533	Pregnant women PW2 (2006) n=515
in Maela [years]	7.0 [0.6 - 18]	7.0 [0.1 - 20]	8.0 [0.3 – 19]
in Thailand [years]	10.0 [0.6 - 30]	10.0 [0.1 - 35]	10.0 [0.5 - 29]
Smokers [% (n)]	28 (25)	28 (150)	27 (138)
Daily betel nut [% (n)] [2]	24 (21)	20 (105) [b]	28 (142)
Nya-u htee per day	2 [0 - 3]	2 [0 - 3]	2 [0 - 3]
2-3x nya-u htee[ny] [% n]	63 (55)	57 (302)	55 (281)
Religion			
Buddhist [% (n)]	43 (38)	43 (226)	47 (243)
Christian [% (n)]	44 (39)	40 (216)	36 (186)
Muslim [% (n)]	12 (11)	17 (90)	16 (84)
Others [% (n)]	1.1 (1)	0.2 (1)	0.4 (2)
Garden, animals			
Own garden [% (n)] [2]	47 (42)	47 (248) [c]	39 (203)
Chicken/ducks [% (n)] [2]	23 (20) [a]	20 (106) [a]	6 (32)
Pigs, goats [% (n)] [2]	13 (12) [a]	18 (95) [a]	30 (157)

Figures are median [range] and percentages (n) ; [ny] 2 to 3 times nya-u htee per day (fermented fish); [2] PW2 different to respective other groups: [a] p<0.001, [b] p<0.01, [c] p<0.05 (p=0.014)

32

The comparison of religion groups revealed that Buddhists had a significantly higher proportion of smokers than Christians and Muslims and more women who chewed daily betel nut than Christians. Muslims consumed significantly less nya-u htee (2-3x per day) than the respective other groups (**Table 3.1.3**). Christians stayed longer in Thailand and in Maela camp and had more frequently their own garden than Buddhists and Muslims. Buddhists households had less often own chicken or ducks and only 4 Muslim women reported having pigs or goats.

Table 3.1.3 Characteristics and life style by religion groups

Characteristics at first ANC consultation	Buddhists n=507 (45%)	Christians n=441 (39%)	Muslims n=185 (16%)
Age [years]	26.0 (20.1-34)	25.8 (20.1-33)	25.3 (19.8-32)
Height [cm] [B]	150.5 (5.3)	151.5 (5.4) [b]	152.1 (5.5) [b]
Weight, T1 [kg] [B]	46.7 (41-53)	47.6 (42-55) [c]	49.0 (41-59) [b]
BMI T1 [kg/m^2] [B]	20.7 (18.5-23)	20.8 (18.3-23.5)	21.2 (18-25) [c]
BMI < 18.5 [% (n)]	15 (76)	17 (74)	19.5 (36)
BMI ≥ 23 [% (n)] [M]	15 (77) [a]	18 (78) [b]	29 (53)
Parity [babies born]	2 [0 - 11]	2 [0 - 9]	2 [0 - 9]
Parity 0 [% (n)]	23 (115)	24 (106)	20 (37)
Parity 1 [% (n)]	21 (104)	25 (112)	24 (44)
Parity 2-3 [% (n)]	33 (169)	33 (144)	28 (52)
Parity ≥ 4 [% (n)] [C]	24 (119) [c]	18 (79)	28 (52) [b]
in Thailand [years] [C]	8.6 (3.7-15.7) [a]	11.6 (5.6-19.7)	8.6 (4.1-14.7) [a]
in Maela [years] [C]	6.4 (3.1-10.8) [a]	7.5 (3.8-12.5)	6.7 (3.7-10.7) [c]
Smokers [% (n)] [B (C)]	36 (184)	24 (106) [a]	11 (21) [a]
Daily betel nut [% (n)] [B]	27 (138)	19.5 (86) [b]	24 (44)
Nya-u htee per day [M]	1.9 (0.8-2.5) [a]	1.8 (0.7-2.5) [a]	0.7 (0-1.4)
2-3x nya-u htee[ny] [% (n)] [M]	67 (338) [a]	64 (281) [a]	9 (17)
Garden, animals			
Own garden [% (n)] [C (B)]	41% (208) [a]	53% (236)	26% (48) [a]
Chicken/ducks [% (n)] [B]	11% (56)	16% (72) [c]	16% (30) [d]
Pigs, goats [% (n)] [M]	26% (134) [a]	29% (126) [a]	2% (4)

Figures are geometric mean (2SD range), mean(SD), median [range] and percentages (n)
[ny] nya-u htee: fermented fish paste; 2-3x nya-u htee: 2 to 3 times daily nya-u htee with the meals
[B] Buddhists, [M] Muslims, [C] Christians significant different (2-sided) to respective other religion group:
[a] p<0.001, [b] p<0.01, [c] p<0.05, ([d] p<0.1)

The comparison between post partum groups (**Table 3.1.4**) revealed that women in the PP group had a lower mean height than those of PP1 and PP2 and a significantly lower mean weight than women of PP1. The proportion of women in PP2 who consumed betel was higher than in PP1. Again, in 2006 the frequency of women reporting to have own chicken or ducks (PP2) was significantly lower whereas the proportion of women reporting to breed pigs or goats was significantly higher than in 2004 (PP, PP1). Further in 2006 the proportion of Buddhists increased while that of Christians simultaneously decreased in comparison to 2004 for both pregnant and post partum groups.

Table 3.1.4 Characteristics and life style by post partum groups (PP, PP1, PP2)

Characteristics in post partum	PP (2004) n=89	PP1 (2004) n=100	PP2 (2006/7) n=474
Age [years]	25.3 (19.7-32.4)	25.6 (19.9-32.9)	26.0 (20.0-33.8)
Height [cm] [0]	149.0 (5.1)	151.1 (4.8) [c]	150.6 (5.3) [c]
Weight [kg] [0]	47.7 (41.5-54.8)	50.3 (44.0-57.6) [c]	49.4 (42.6-57.2)
BMI	21.5 (19.1-24.2)	22.1 (19.6-24.9)	21.8 (19.2-24.7)
BMI < 18.5 [% (n)]	7 (6)	5 (5)	8 (39)
BMI ≥ 23 [% (n)]	27 (24)	35 (35)	30 (140)
Parity [babies born]	3 [1 - 9]	3 [1 - 10]	3 [1 - 10]
Smokers [% (n)]	28 (25)	32 (32)	26 (121)
Daily betel nut [% (n)] [2]	24 (21)	19 (19) [d]	27 (130)
Nya-u htee per day	2 [0 - 3]	2 [0 - 3]	2 [0 - 3]
2-3x nya-u htee /d [% n]	63 (55)	62 (62)	55 (259)
Religion			
Buddhist [% (n)]	43 (38)	38 (38)	46 (217)
Christian [% (n)]	44 (39)	45 (45)	37 (177)
Muslim [% (n)]	12 (11)	17 (17)	17 (80)
Others [% (n)]	1.1 (1)	0	0
Garden, animals			
Own garden [% (n)]	47 (42)	47 (47)	38 (181)
Chicken, ducks [% (n)] [2]	23 (20) [a]	12 (12) [c]	6 (29)
Pigs, goats [% (n)] [2]	14 (12) [a]	13 (13) [a]	31 (145)

Figures are geometric mean (2SD range), mean(SD), median [range] and percentages (n)
[0] PP , [2] PP2 group different to respective other groups: [a] $p<0.001$, [b] $p<0.01$, [c] $p<0.05$, ([d] $p<0.1$)

3.2 Flow chart of collected samples for biochemical measurements

Numbers of blood and milk samples collected between March 2004 and September 2007 as well as available valid birth weights, separated by different pregnant and post partum groups, are summarized in **Table 3.2**. Serum and whole blood were available from all women and breast milk samples from women in post partum. Of the 533 pregnant women in PW1, 67 were in trimester 1, 250 in trimester 2 (13-26 wks), and 216 in trimester 3 ($\geq$ 27 wks); the second cross-sectional survey (PW2) revealed a similar proportion with 52, 217 and 246 women in trimester 1, 2 and 3, respectively. Pregnant women of PW1 and PW2, separated by trimester, were compared to mothers in 12 weeks post partum (PP). A cohort of 100 women from PW1 (PP1) who were for the first time provided with the micronutrient enriched flour (lactational MEF) and a second cohort of 470 women (PP2) who received the micronutrient enriched flour during pregnancy as well as in post partum (pregnancy and lactational MEF) were compared with the post partum women (PP) who never received the flour.

Table 3.2 Flow chart on number of collected samples and 'valid' birth weights

Time period of sampling	Group (N)	(T) Tri-mester	N blood samples	N Birth weights	N blood and milk samples
March - April 2004	PP (89)			87	
June - July 2004					89 PP No MEF
Rainy season June - July 2004	PW1 (533)	T1 T2 T3	67 250 216		
June 04 - Jan 05				501	
Sept - Nov 2004				→	100 PP1 Lactational MEF
November 2006 *Dry season*	PW2 (515)	T1 T2 T3	52 217 246		
Dec 06 - June 07				489	
Feb - Sept 2007				→	470 PP2 Pregnancy and Lactational MEF

3.3 Impact by infections markers C-reactive protein (CRP) and α-1glycoproteine (AGP) on blood micronutrients in pregnancy and post partum

Pregnant women had higher mean CRP and higher proportion of elevated levels (CRP >5 mg/L) than post partum women. There was no significant trend of CRP by trimester of pregnancy. Second trimester women of PW2 (2006) had a significant higher CRP and AGP (2.15 vs. 1.44 mg/L and 0.48 vs. 0.44 g/L) than women of PW1 (2004). Increased AGP (>1g/L) was only relevant in trimester 1 with a similar proportion as in post partum women. In post partum women PP2 had a higher mean CRP but lower mean AGP than PP1 and PP, but proportions of elevated CRP or AGP didn't differ between post partum groups. Blood samples of pregnant and post partum women with CRP > 5mg/L and APG > 1g/L showed significantly lower serum retinol and β-carotene but significantly higher serum ferritin and copper than those with CRP < 5mg/L and AGP < 1g/L. However, micronutrient levels were not adjusted for high CRP or AGP, and all cases were included in statistical analysis. CRP (>5mg/L=1) and AGP (>1g/L=1) were used as binary variables in linear and logistic regression analysis assessing predictors for micronutrient concentrations and respective deficiencies. Less than 2% of pregnant women (18/1,046) and none of post partum women had an acute malaria episode at blood draw. 15 women were infected with *P. vivax* and 3 women had an episode from *P. falciparum*. Acute respiratory and urinary tract infections (20x) and vaginal and skin diseases (25x) including scabies and abscesses were the most frequent morbid events beside malaria at time of sample collection.

Table 3.3 CRP and AGP by trimester of pregnancy and post partum groups [**]

Trimester, T	T1, n=118	T2, n=466	T3, n=462
CRP [mg/L]	1.03 (0.17-6.15)	1.74 (0.44-6.82)	1.46 (0.38-5.66)
% (n) > 5 mg/L	20 (23)	21 (96)	18 (81)
AGP [g/L] [1a]	0.714 (0.51-1.01)	0.459 (0.32-0.67)	0.413 (0.29-0.59)
% (n) > 1 g/L	14 (17)	2 (8)	1 (4)
Post partum, PP	**PP, n=89**	**PP1, n=99**	**PP2, n=470**
CRP [mg/L] [2]	0.317 [c] (0.04-2.69)	0.317 [c] (0.04-2.35)	0.552 (0.10-2.95)
% (n) > 5 mg/L	7 (6)	6 (6)	10 (46)
AGP [g/L] [2]	0.784 [b] (0.55-1.06)	0.747 [b] (0.57-0.95)	0.680 (0.44-0.98)
% (n) > 1 g/L	17 (15)	14 (14)	13 (59)

[**] Figures are geometric mean (2SD range: -/+ 1 SD), and percentage (n)
[1] Trimester trend (linear regression), [2] PP2 different to PP1 and PP: [a] $p < 0.001$, [b] $p < 0.01$, [c] $p < 0.05$

3.4 Fat soluble vitamins in serum and breast-milk

Serum concentrations of retinol, β-carotene, and α-tocopherol as well as of cholesterol and triglycerides in pregnant and postpartum women are shown in **Table 3.4.1** and **Fig. 3.4.1**. Retinol is lower whereas β-carotene, α-tocopherol and serum triglycerides were higher in pregnant than in post partum women. α-Tocopherol, cholesterol and triglycerides increased significantly whereas retinol and β-carotene decreased with increasing trimester. All fat soluble vitamins were significantly positive correlated with each other (Pearson, p<0.001), with cholesterol, and except for β-carotene with triglycerides during pregnancy and post partum (**Tables 3.4.2a-c**). The significant increase of α-tocopherol from 1st to 3rd trimester is most likely caused by the simultaneously increase of cholesterol and triglycerides.

Table 3.4.1 Fat soluble vitamins in serum during pregnancy and post partum [**]

Serum vitamins [μmol/L]	Trimester 1 (5,3 - 12,6)[*] n=118	Trimester 2 (13,0 - 26,6)[*] n=466	Trimester 3 (27,0 - 40,5)[*] n=462	mothers PP week 12 n=89
Retinol [1c, 2a]	1.32 (0.32)	1.42 (0.37)	1.30 (0.4)	1.60 (0.4)
< 1.05 μmol/L	23%	14%	27%	6%
α-Tocopherol [1a, 2a]	16.3 (3.9)	21.3 (5.4)	27.0 (6.5)	13.4 (3.8)
< 11.6 μmol/L	8%	3%	<0.5%	33%
β-Carotene [1c, 2b]	0.235 (0.13-0.424)	0.231 (0.128-0.420)	0.209 (0.103-0.422)	0.179 (0.085-0.377)
< 0.3 μmol/L	64%	68%	70%	74%
Cholesterol [1a, 2a] [mmol/L]	3.78 (3.10-4.53)	4.65 (3.69-5.72)	5.74 (4.57-7.05)	4.60 (3.76-5.52)
Triglycerides [1a, 2c] [mmol/L]	1.19 (0.74-1.75)	2.04 (1.32-2.91)	3.05 (2.05-4.24)	1.05 (0.58-1.65)
α-Tocopherol / total serum fat [μmol/g] [2a]	3.20 (0.53)	3.21 (0.57)	3.16 (0.55)	2.40 (0.44)

[*] Gestational age at blood draw (weeks,days), [**] Figures are mean (SD), geometric mean (2SD range)
[1] Trimester trend (linear regression): [a] p < 0.001, [b] p < 0.01, [c] p < 0.05
[2] Post partum group (PP) vs. Trimester 1: [a] p < 0.001, [b] p < 0.01, [c] p < 0.05

Once adjusted for total serum fat (sum of cholesterol, triglycerides and phospho-lipids), α-tocopherol did not vary between trimester and was used as a proxy for gestational age adjusted α-tocopherol in analysis assessing pregnancy outcomes.

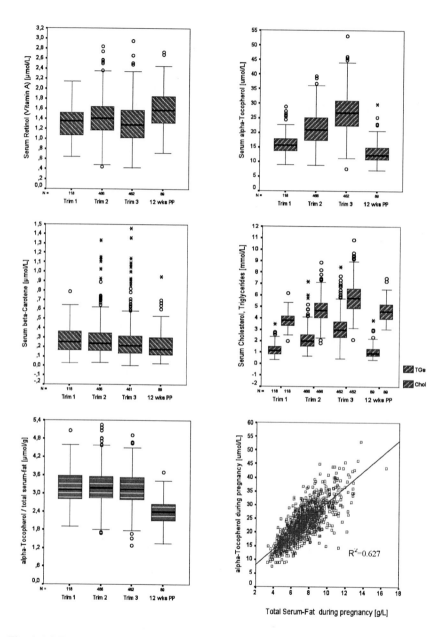

Fig. 3.4.1 Fat soluble vitamins by trimesters of pregnancy and in post partum

Tables 3.4.2a-c: Linear regression analysis on predictors of fat soluble vitamin

a. Serum retinol [μmol/L] in pregnancy, n=1046 (Adj. R^2=17%)

	B	S. E.	Beta	t	Sig.	Adj. R^2
(Constant)	1,421	,068		20,96	,000	
Triglycerides [mmol/L]	,105	,012	,321	8,64	,000	,027
EGA at blood draw [weeks]	-,016	,002	-,363	-9,06	,000	,076
Sample 2004 [=1], 2006 [=2]	-,149	,022	-,195	-6,82	,000	,106
AGP > 1 g/L (=1)	-,313	,069	-,135	-4,56	,000	,135
CRP > 5 mg/L (=1)	-,125	,028	-,128	-4,41	,000	,152
Cholesterol [mmol/L]	,041	,011	,139	3,85	,000	,163
Age at admission [years]	,004	,002	,074	2,57	,010	**,168**

b. Predictors of serum α-tocopherol [μmol/L] in pregnancy, n=1044 (Adj. R^2=68%)

	B	S. E.	Beta	t	Sig.	Adj R^2
(Constant)	2,066	,583		3,54	,000	
Cholesterol s1 [mmol/L]	3,124	,106	,592	29,34	,000	**,588**
Triglycerides [mmol/L]	1,955	,118	,334	16,56	,000	**,667**
Smoking [yes=1]	-1,241	,282	-,081	-4,41	,000	,676
Sample 2004 [=1], 2006 [=2]	,787	,241	,058	3,26	,001	,679
Parity [N babies born]	-,178	,065	-,050	-2,73	,007	,681

c. Predictors of β-carotene [log e μmol/L] in pregnancy, n=1045 (Adj. R^2=15.2%)

	B	S. E.	Beta	t	Sig.	Adj. R^2
(Constant)	-1,580	,093		-17,02	,000	
Cholesterol s1 (mmol/L)	,201	,018	,403	11,09	,000	,037
EGA at blood draw [weeks]	-,017	,003	-,240	-5,95	,000	,098
Triglycerides [mmol/L]	-,087	,021	-,156	-4,18	,000	,117
AGP > 1 g/L (=1)	-,379	,117	-,096	-3,23	,001	,129
Parity (babies born)	-,035	,010	-,105	-3,64	,000	,139
Sample 2004 (1) 2007 (2)	-,132	,037	-,102	-3,54	,000	,148
CRP > 5 mg/L (=1)	-,117	,048	-,071	-2,42	,016	,152

The main predictors for high concentrations of fat soluble vitamins in pregnancy were serum triglycerides, cholesterol, acute phase proteins (CRP, AGP) and year of sampling (**Tables 3.4.2a-c**). All fat soluble vitamins were positively correlated with serum cholesterol. Retinol and α-tocopherol were highly positively while β-carotene was negatively associated with serum triglycerides. The increase and positive association with both serum cholesterol and triglycerides explained 67% of the variation in serum α-tocopherol (**Table 3.4.2b, Fig. 3.4.1**). Retinol and β-carotene were significantly lower whereas α-tocopherol, serum fat (cholesterol, triglycerides) and fat adjusted α-tocopherol were significantly higher in 2006 than in the year 2004. Elevated acute phase proteins (CRP, AGP) were negatively associated with retinol and β-carotene. Additionally, smoking and the consumption of nya-u htee became significant factors when included in the models for fat soluble vitamins: Women who smoked had significantly higher retinol but lower α-tocopherol and β-carotene, and the frequent consumption of nya-u thee (2-3x per day) was positively associated with retinol and β-carotene but inversely correlated with α-tocopherol. Furthermore, having a garden was associated with higher serum β-carotene. Smoking, nya-u htee consumption, and having a garden are life style factors which showed a strong association with reported religious group: Muslims, who consumed nya-u htee less often (< 10% vs. 67% of Buddhists and 64% of Christians), who had the lowest proportion in smokers (11% vs. 36% of Buddhists and 24% Christians) and who less often reported having their own garden (26% vs. 41% of Buddhists and 53% of Christians), had significantly lower mean serum retinol and β-carotene (1.22 and 0.164 µmol/L) than Buddhists (1.37 and 0.218 µmol/L, p<0.001) and Christians (1.41 and 0.258 µmol/L, p<0.001). Buddhists, who had the highest proportion of smokers and nya-u htee consumers, had a significantly lower mean α-tocopherol than Christians (22.6 vs. 23.9 µmol/L) as well as a significantly lower fat adjusted α-tocopherol than Muslims (3.1 vs. 3.33 µmol/g). Christians with the highest proportion in women who reported to have an own garden and pigs or goats had highest mean values of both serum β-carotene and retinol. Further households who had their own garden had significantly more frequently chicken (17 vs. 10%) and pigs or goats (30 vs. 20%) than those who had not.

In summary Christian was a positive whereas Muslim was a negative predictor for serum retinol and β-carotene. Muslim was a positive while Buddhist was a negative predictor for α-tocopherol. Religious groups replaced smoking and nya-u htee consumption as significant predictors in multivariate models. However, the main predictor for serum β-carotene beside serum fat was of course the availability of fruits and vegetables and therefore the respective season at blood draw.

Risk factors for a low serum retinol during pregnancy (< 1.05 µmol/L, **Table 3.4.3**) agreed well with the predictors for serum retinol obtained by linear regression analysis: increasing gestational age or 3rd compared to 1st trimester at blood draw, high CRP, to be Muslim compared to be Christian, blood collected in 2006 vs. 2004, and an elevated AGP increased the risk by 3.5, 2.1, 2.3, 1.7 and 3.4 fold, respectively; whereas high serum triglycerides and smoking decreased the risk for low serum retinol. Smoking reduced the risk for vitamin A deficiency most likely due to its association with age and religious group: mean age of smokers was significantly higher (29.9 vs. 25.4 years, p<0.001) than of non-smokers and 92% of the smokers were not Muslim (either Buddhists 59% or Christian) 33%).

Table 3.4.3 Risk factors for retinol <1.05 µmol/L in pregnancy, n=220/1043 (21%)

	B	S. E.	Wald	Sig.	Exp(B)	95% C.I.	
Constant	-2,044	,394	26,966	,000	,129		
Trimester 1 (control)			45,301	,000	control		
Trimester 2	-,068	,294	,053	,818	,935	,526	1,662
Trimester 3	1,265	,320	15,647	,000	**3,54**	1,893	6,635
Triglycerides [mmol/L]	-,434	,094	21,268	,000	,65	,539	,779
CRP > 5 mg/L (=1)	,745	,196	14,489	,000	2,11	1,435	3,091
Christians (control; n=401)			13,352	,001	control		
Bhuddists (=1; n=469)	,360	,188	3,666	,056	1,43	,992	2,070
Muslims (=1; n=173)	,822	,225	13,293	,000	**2,28**	1,462	3,538
Year 2004 (=1) 2007 (=2)	,509	,164	9,650	,002	1,66	1,207	2,295
Smoking (yes=1)	-,575	,205	7,908	,005	,56	,377	,840
AGP > 1 g/L (=1)	1,194	,446	7,154	,007	**3,30**	1,376	7,913

The comparison of fat soluble vitamin levels between the post partum groups (**Table 3.4.4**) showed highest mean serum retinol in PP1 and highest mean α-tocopherol, β-carotene and triglycerides in PP2.

**Table 3.4.4 Fat soluble vitamins in post partum (PP) groups [**]

Fat soluble vitamins [µmol/L]	PP 2004 n=89	PP1 2004 n=99	PP2 2007 n=470
Retinol [2(07c)]	1.60 (0.4)	1.69 (0.46)[c]	1.57 (0.45)
%(n)< 1.05 µmol/L [(07c)]	6 (5)	6 (6)	11 (51)
α-Tocopherol [2(07a)]	13.1[a] (9.85-16.9)	14.1[b] (10.3-18.5)	15.5 (11.4-20.1)
%(n)<11.6 µmol/L [2(07b)]	33[a] (29)	23 (23)	16 (76)
β-Carotene [2(07a)]	0.179[c] (0.085-0.377)	0.167[a] (0.089-0.312)	0.217 (0.117-0.401)
%(n)< 0.3 µmol/L [2(07b)]	74 (6)	83[b] (82)	68 (318)
Cholesterol [mmol/L]	4.56 (3.77-5.51)	4.72 (3.84-5.80)	4.56 (3.66-5.67)
Triglycerides [2(07c)] [mmol/L]	0.98[c] (0.60-1.60)	1.02 (0.64-1.62)	1.10 (0.68-1.79)
α-Tocopherol / serum fat [µmol/g] [2(07a)]	2.40 (0.44)[a]	2.50 (0.48)[a]	2.77 (0.58)

[**] Figures are mean (SD), geometric mean (2SD range: -/+ 1 SD), and percentages
[2] PP2 different to respective other groups: [a] p< 0.001, [b] p< 0.01, [c] p< 0.05
[(07)] Year 2007 (PP2) different to year 2004 (PP2 vs. PP1-PP): [a] p< 0.001, [b] p< 0.01, [c] p< 0.05

Predictors for fat soluble vitamins in the post partum period by linear regression analysis (**Tables 3.4.5a-d**) are in agreement with those shown for pregnant women. Serum cholesterol as the main predictor was highly positive associated with all fat soluble vitamins. Serum triglycerides were positive associated with retinol and α-tocopherol but inversely correlated with β-carotene. Again, serum retinol was significantly lower whereas α-tocopherol, fat adjusted α-tocopherol, and triglycerides were significantly higher in 2007 (PP 2) than in 2004 (PP, PP1). Smoking and to be Buddhist was negatively, whereas to be Muslim, was positively associated with α-tocopherol. To be Buddhist or have high consumption of nya-u htee was positively whereas elevated CRP or AGP and to be Muslim was negatively associated with serum retinol and β-carotene.

Table 3.4.5a-d: Linear regression analysis on fat soluble vitamin in serum

a. Predicors of serum retinol in post partum [μmol/L], n=658 (R^2=28%)

	B	S. E.	Beta	t	Sig.	Adj. R^2
(Constant)	,712	,123		5,81	,000	
Cholesterol s2 [mmol/L]	,135	,017	,304	7,89	,000	,173
Triglyceride s2 [mmol/L]	,163	,027	,240	6,13	,000	,229
Age at admission [years]	,009	,002	,144	3,86	,000	,244
CRP > 5 mg/L (=1)	-,175	,057	-,111	-3,09	,002	,260
Sample 2004 [=1], 2007 [=2]	-,124	,043	-,103	-2,86	,004	,269
Buddhist (=1)	,080	,033	,088	2,45	,015	,277

b. Predictors of α-tocopherol in post partum [√ μmol/L], n=658 (R^2=54%)

	B	S. E.	Beta	t	Sig.	Adj. R^2
(Constant)	1,716	,092		18,61	,000	
Cholesterol pp [mmol/L]	,330	,016	,598	20,95	,000	,431
sample bw 2004 (1) 2007 (2)	,235	,033	,191	7,169	,000	,478
Triglyceride pp [mmol/L]	,177	,024	,211	7,27	,000	,511
Smoking [yes=1]	-,147	,034	-,117	-4,30	,000	,528
Muslim (=1)	,161	,040	,108	3,99	,000	,539

c. Predictors of serum β-carotene [log e μmol/L] in post partum, n=658

	B	S. E.	Beta	t	Sig.	Adj. R^2
(Constant)	-2,808	,143		-19,62	,000	
Cholesterol pp [mmol/L]	,205	,024	,320	8,36	,000	,091
Muslim (=1)	-,305	,063	-,176	-4,88	,000	,127
Sample 2004 [=1], 2007 [=2]	,249	,051	,175	4,89	,000	,156
AGP > 1 g/L (=1)	-,212	,068	-,112	-3,11	,002	,168
Triglyceride pp [mmol/L]	-,077	,037	-,079	-2,05	,040	,172

Paired samples t-tests in the follow-up groups (PP1, PP2) revealed that fat soluble vitamins (retinol, α-tocopherol, β-carotene), serum lipids (cholesterol, triglycerides, total fat) and lipid adjusted α-tocopherol in pregnancy were significantly positively correlated with respective levels in week 12 post partum. Therefore, women who had a vitamin deficiency during pregnancy were at high risk to be still deficient in the respective vitamin at 12 weeks post partum. Retinol levels in pregnancy explained 19% of the variance in serum retinol in post partum (**Table 3.4.5d**).

d. Predictors of serum retinol [μmol/L] in post partum n=569 (R^2=39.6%)

	B	S. E.	Beta	t	Sig.	Adj. R^2
(Constant)	,242	,120		2,01	,045	
retinol in pregnancy [μmol/L]	,444	,041	,356	10,73	,000	**,190**
Cholesterol pp [mmol/L]	,122	,016	,274	7,79	,000	,327
Triglyceride pp [mmol/L]	,148	,024	,217	6,09	,000	,369
CRP > 5 mg/L (=1)	-,160	,052	-,101	-3,08	,002	,378
Age at admission [years]	,007	,002	,108	3,17	,002	,386
Sample 2004 [=1], 2007 [=2]	-,101	,039	-,084	-2,56	,011	,391
Buddhist (=1)	,069	,030	,075	2,30	,022	,396

Concentrations of fat soluble vitamins in breast milk by post partum groups are provided in **Table 3.4.6**. Retinol, α-tocopherol, β-carotene and other carotenoids (lutein, zeaxanthin, β-cryptoxanthin) per milk volume [μmol/L] were significantly higher in 2007 (PP2) than in 2004 (PP, PP1). Retinol, α-tocopherol and β-carotene in breast milk were strongly affected by the milk fat concentration and respective vitamin levels in serum (**Table 3.4.7a-c; Fig. 3.4.2**). Overall, correlations between fat soluble vitamins in milk and serum improved after adjustment for milk fat. Breast milk levels of lutein-zeaxanthin (per volume and fat adjusted) were significantly higher (>3 fold) than those of β-carotene and β-cryptoxanthin. Milk fat adjusted retinol, lutein-zeaxanthin and β-cryptoxanthin didn't differ between post partum groups or year of sampling whereas fat adjusted α-tocopherol and β-carotene were still significantly higher in 2007 than in 2004. The high proportion of low retinol per milk volume (<1.05 μmol/L) with 35% (28-53%) decreased considerably to 12% (4.5-17%) of low or deficient retinol levels after adjustment for milk fat (<28 μmol/kg fat) and was significantly lower in the first post partum group (PP) in 2004.

Table 3.4.6 Fat soluble vitamins in breast milk

Vitamins and fat in breast milk [**]	PP, 2004 n=88	PP 1, 2004 n=96	PP2, 2007 n=460
Retinol [µmol/L] [2, 07a]	1.09 [a] (0.64-1.66)	1.01 [a] (0.54-1.61)	1.36 (0.80-2.06)
% (n)< 1.05 µmol/L [2]	51 [a] (45)	53 [a] (51)	28 (128)
α-Tocopherol [2, 07a] [µmol/L]	3.68 [a] (2.08-5.74)	3.50 [a] (1.99-2.33)	5.01 (3.07-7.44)
β-Carotene [2, 07a] [µmol/L]	0.014 [a] (79) (0.006-0.029)	0.010 [a] (83) (0.005-0.017)	0.025 (454) (0.012-0.052)
Lutein-zeaxanthin [2, 07a] [µmol/L]	0.074 [c] (0.04-0.138)	0.071 [b] (0.04-0.129)	0.088 (0.053-0.144)
β-Cryptoxanthin [2, 07a] [µmol/L]	0.011 [a] (83) (0.006-0.022)	0.010 [a] (92) (0.005-0.022)	0.016 (443) (0.007-0.034)
Milk fat [g/L] [2, 07a]	24.2 [a] (10.4)	23.8 [a] (9.4)	31.3 (11.8)
Retinol / fat	46.9 (33.9-65.0)	43.0 (27.2-68.0)	44.4 (29.9-65.9)
% (n)< 28 µmol/kg [2]	4.5 (4) [c]	17 (16)	12 (54)
α-Tocopherol / fat [2, 07c] [µmol/kg]	156.7 (107.0-229.4)	150.3 [c] (103.7-217.8)	164.6 (112.9-240.1)
β-Carotene / fat [2 (1)] [µmol/kg] [(p/y-a)]	0.595 [a] (79) (0.286-1.238)	0.427 [a] (83) (0.250-0.728)	0.861 (454) (0.431-1.718)
Lutein-zeaxanthin / fat [µmol/kg]	3.38 (1.84-6.22)	3.26 (1.67-6.37)	3.03 (1.76-5.19)
Cryptoxanthin / fat [(2)] [µmol/L]	0.507 (83) (0.257-1.00)	0.457 [d] (92) (0.235-0.887)	0.536 (443) (0.254-1.13)

[**] Figures are mean (SD), geometric mean (2SD range: -/+ 1 SD), and percentages
[2] PP2 different to PP1 and/or PP, [(1)] PP1 different to PP: [a] $p < 0.001$, [b] $p < 0.01$, [c] $p < 0.05$, ([d] $p < 0.06$)
[07] year 2007 (PP2) different to 2004 (PP, PP1): [a] $p < 0.001$, [b] $p < 0.01$, [c] $p < 0.05$

Table 3.4.7a-c Predictors of fat soluble vitamins in breast milk

a. Retinol in breast milk [$\sqrt{}$ µmol/L], n=639 (R^2=34%)

	B	S. E.	Beta	t	Sig.	Adj. R^2
(Constant)	,464	,052		8,97	,000	
Milk fat g/L	,012	,001	,530	15,74	,000	,292
Serum Retinol pp [µmol/L]	,125	,020	,199	6,11	,000	,327
Sample 2004 [=1], 2007 [=2]	,061	,020	,101	2,99	,003	,336

b. α-Tocopherol in breast milk [$\sqrt{}$ µmol/L], n=638 (R^2=42%)

	B	S. E.	Beta	t	Sig.	Adj. R^2
(Constant)	,144	,151		,955	,340	
Milk fat g/L	,024	,001	,555	17,69	,000	,351
Serum α-Tocopherol / fat in post partum [$\sqrt{}$ µmol/g]	,689	,093	,231	7,40	,000	,414
Sample 2004 [=1], 2007 [=2]	,106	,036	,094	2,91	,004	,420

<u>c. β-Carotene in breast milk [log e μmol/L], n=612 (R^2=57%)</u>

	B	S. E.	Beta	t	Sig.	Adj. R^2
(Constant)	-4,330	,110		-39,19	,000	
Serum β-carotene in post partum [log e μmol/L]	,714	,034	,558	20,77	,000	**,326**
Milk fat [g/L]	,024	,002	,353	12,84	,000	,501
Sample 2004 [=1], 2007 [=2]	,484	,050	,270	9,78	,000	,568

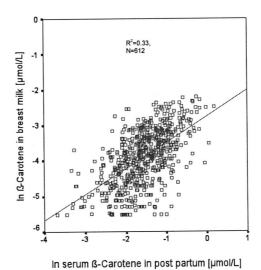

ln serum ß-Carotene in post partum [μmol/L]

Fig. 3.4.2 Impact of serum β-carotene on β-carotene levels in breast milk

45

3.5 Thiamine in whole blood and breast milk

Thiamine di-phosphate (TDP) per volume of whole blood [µg/L] and adjusted for hemoglobin [ng/g] is shown in Table **3.5.1**. TDP increased during pregnancy (from 1st to 3rd trimester) and was significantly higher in post-partum than in trimester 1. Betel nut consumption and smoking was associated with significant lower TDP in 3rd trimester. Multiple regression analysis revealed that higher hemoglobin, older age and an increased number of days receiving B1 supplements were positive, while to be Buddhist and smoking, were negative predictors for whole blood TDP during pregnancy; whilst in the post partum period higher hemoglobin, to be Christian and older age were positive predictors and blood samples collected in 2007 was a negative determinant of whole blood TDP (**Table 3.5.2 a-b**)

Table 3.5.1 Whole blood thiamine di-phosphate in pregnancy and post partum

Thiamine (TDP) in whole blood and per hemoglobin	Trimester 1 $(5,3 - 12,6)^g$ n=118	Trimester 2 $(13,0 - 26,6)^g$ n=467	Trimester 3 $(27,0 - 40,5)^g$ n=462	mothers PP week 12 n=89
TDP [µg/L] [1c, 2a]	48.3 (32.6 - 67.2)	50.4 (34.3 - 69.6)	51.1 (33.5 - 72.3)	65.2 (44.9 - 89.4)
< 30 µg/L (< 65 nM)	13% (n=15)	9.4% (n=44)	11% (n=49)	3.4% (n=3)
TDP [nmol/L] [1c, 2a]	104.9 (70.7 - 145.8)	109.5 (74.5 - 151.1)	110.9 (72.6 - 157)	141.6 (97.4 - 194)
Hb [2a]	115.5 (10.9)	108.2 (11.2)	108.3 (11.6)	124.7 (10.9)
TDP / Hb [2a] [ng/g]	420.9 (282 - 588)	470.1 (318 - 652)	473.5 (313 - 667)	526.5 (361 - 723)
B1 supplements [B1S] [weeks] [1a, 2a]	2 [0-8]	9 [0-25]	20 [0-34]	40 [13-47]
TDP daily betel vs. [3b] seldom/no betel [µg/L]	47.0 (n=29) 48.8 (n=89)	49.4 (n=118) 50.8 (n=347)	46.3 (n=100) [b] 52.4 (n=367) [b]	64.7 (n=21) 65.4 (n=68)
TDP smoker vs. [3b] non-smoker [µg/L]	49.3 (n=38) 47.9 (n=80)	48.9 (n=124) 51.0 (n=341)	46.1 (n=126) [b] 53.0 (n=336) [b]	61.4 (n=25) 66.8 (n=64)

Figures are geometric mean (2SD range: -/+ 1 SD), mean (SD) and median [range]
TDP: thiamine diphosphate ; Hb: hemoglobin (estimated by hematocrit: x 3.33)
[g] Gestational age at blood draw (weeks), [B1S] weeks of provided vitamin B1 (thiamine mono-sulphate)
[1] Trimester trend (linear regression), [2] Post partum vs. Trimester 1, [a] $p < 0.001$, [b] $p < 0.01$, [c] $p < 0.05$
[3] Difference between betel nut consumer or smoker vs. seldom/no betel or non-smoker: [b] $p<0.01$

The proportion of betel nut consumers was highest in the group of Buddhists and was significantly higher in smokers than in non-smokers (46% in smokers vs. 15% in non-smokers, p<0.001); further women who smoked or consumed daily betel had significantly lower hemoglobin during pregnancy than those who did not (106 and 104 g/L vs. 109 and 110 g/L, respectively). Maximum TDP levels in each trimester and in post partum groups were found in the non-smokers and those who never or seldom consumed betel, whereas lowest TDP levels were detected in each subgroup including the non-smokers or those who never chewed betel nut. Smoking as well as betel nut consumption was inversely associated with hemoglobin which was highly predictive of TDP in pregnancy and in the post partum period (**Table 3.5.2 a-b**).

Table 3.5.2 Predictors for Thiamine diphosphate (TDP) in whole blood

a. Thiamine di phosphate in pregnancy [√ µg/L], n=1044

	B	S. E.	Beta	t	Sig.	Adj. R^2
(Constant)	4,710	,422		11,17	,000	
Buddhist (=1)	-,455	,078	-,175	-5,80	,000	,037
Hemoglobin [g/L]	,016	,003	,140	4,64	,000	,051
Age at admission	,028	,006	,148	4,76	,000	,064
Provided B1 supplements [weeks]	,017	,005	,111	3,70	,000	,076
Smoking [yes=1]	-,270	,091	-,093	-2,95	,003	,083

b. Thiamine di phosphate in post partum [√ µg/L], n=653

	B	S. E.	Beta	t	Sig.	Adj. R^2
(Constant)	8,301	,850		9,77	,000	
Sample 2004 (=1), 2007 (=2)	-1,175	,152	-,283	-7,74	,000	,074
Hemoglobin, pp [g/L]	,031	,006	,182	4,50	,000	,107
Christian (=1)	,535	,139	,140	3,85	,000	,125
Age, adm. [years]	,030	,010	,111	3,05	,002	,136

Post partum women of PP1 who received for the first time the enriched flour had the highest mean levels in whole blood TDP, hemoglobin adjusted TDP as well as in breast milk thiamine. Two years later in 2007, women in post partum (PP2) had significantly lower whole blood TDP and TDP per hemoglobin than those in 2004 (PP, PP1) (**Table 3.5.2b, 3.5.3**). In general, Christians had significantly higher whole blood TDP (61.9 vs. 55.5 and 55.6 µg/L) as well as higher hemoglobin adjusted TDP in post partum than had Buddhists and Muslims (492 vs. 440 and 449 ng/g hemoglobin respectively). In each post partum and religious group whole blood TDP was significantly positively associated with breast milk levels of thiamine (B1), thiamine mono-phosphate (TMP) and total thiamine (TMP + B1): 39% of the variance (Adj. R^2=0,389) in total thiamine in breast milk was explained by whole blood TDP (**Table 3.5.4, Fig 3.5.1**). Christians had significantly higher breast milk thiamine than had Buddhists and Muslim (272 vs. 242 and 246 µg/L). Total thiamine in milk showed considerable variation which ranged between lowest values of 19.3 to highest of 744.6 µg/L (**Fig. 3.5.2**). In 2007, mean total thiamine in breast milk was still as high as in 2004 despite a significantly lower whole blood TDP than in 2004. Overall, less than 5% of the milk samples had levels <100 µg/L, a cut-off indicating low milk thiamine. The amount of thiamine mono-phosphate per total B1 ranged between 4 to 96% with a mean of 61%; therefore mean values of total thiamine consisted of more thiamine mono-phosphate than the non-phosphorylated 'free' thiamine. PP1 with the highest levels in total milk thiamine had significantly higher B1 (thiamine) than the other post partum groups.

Table 3.5.3 Thiamine in whole blood and breast milk by post partum groups

Whole blood	mothers PP 2004 N=89	mothers PP 1 2004 N=100	mothers PP2 2007 N=471
TDP [µg/L] [2]	65.2 [a] (44.9 - 89.4)	68.0 [a] (51.6 - 86.6)	54.7 (38.2 - 74.1)
< 30 µg/L (< 65 nM)	3.4% (n=3)	---	6.6% (n=31)
TDP [nmol/L] [2]	141.6 [a] (97.4 - 194)	147.5 [a] (112 - 188)	118.7 (83 - 161)
Hemoglobin (Hb) [g/L]	124.7 (10.9)	124.4 (9.4)	126.2 (11.2)
TDP / Hb** [2] [ng/g]	526.5 [a] (86) (361 - 723)	546.8 [a] (97) (419 - 692)	434.7 (470) (305 - 587)
Breast milk	N=88	N=98	N=460
TMP [µg/L]	189.5 (110 - 245)	191.0 (134 - 235)	197.5 (127 - 249)
B1 (Thiamine) [µg/L] [1]	78.0[b] (28.3 - 215)	115.5 (60.3 - 221)	79.7[b] (33.6 - 189)
Total Thiamine [µg/L] [1]	245.1 [c] (132 - 393)	279.1 (194 - 379)	250.5 [c] (155 - 369)
Total B1< 100 µg/L	8% (n=7)	2% (n=2)	4% (n=19)
Total Thiamine [1] [nmol/L]	726.7 [c] (391 - 1166)	827.6 (576 - 1124)	742.7 [c] (459 - 1095)
TMP / total B1 [nM%] [1]	64 [c] (44-78) %	57 (39-70) %	65 [c] (46-79) %

Figures are geometric mean (2SD range: -1SD to +1SD) and mean (SD)
*TDP: thiamine diphosphate, TMP: thiamine mono phosphate, B1: thiamine (-chloride)
** Hb: hemoglobin (estimated by hematocrit: x 3.33); Total thiamine: sum of TMP and B1
[1] PP1, [2] PP2 different to respective other post partum groups: [a] p< 0.001, [b] p< 0.01, [c] p< 0.05

Table 3.5.4 Predictors of total thiamine in breast milk [√µg/L], N=643

	B	S. E.	Beta	t	Sig.	Adj. R^2
(Constant)	,706	1,508		,47	,640	
TDP in whole blood [√µg/L]	3,090	,148	,665	20,87	,000	,389
Sample 2004 [=1], 2007 [=2]	1,863	,416	,143	4,48	,000	,407

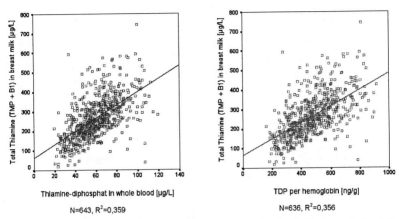

N=643, R^2=0,359   N=636, R^2=0,356

Fig 3.5.1 Association between whole blood thiamine di-phosphate (a) or hemoglobin adjusted TDP (b) and total thiamine in breast milk

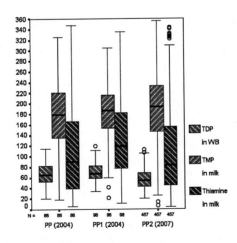

Fig. 3.5.2 Whole blood thiamine (TDP) and its relation to thiamine mono-phosphate (TMP) and thiamine in breast milk by different post partum groups

49

3.6 Iron status, zinc and copper during pregnancy and post partum

Iron status assessed by serum ferritin (SF), soluble transferrin receptor (sTfR) and iron storage (equation using both indicators), hematocrit and serum levels of zinc and copper, during pregnancy and post partum, are given in **Table 3.6.1** and **Fig. 3.6.1**. Serum ferritin (SF) and hematocrit decreased while sTfR and the proportion of iron deficiency (ID) as well as of iron deficiency anemia (IDA) simultaneously increased from 1st to 3rd trimester of pregnancy. SF rose again in post partum women but mean values didn't reach the concentrations found in 1st trimester women. sTfR and the proportion of ID (38%) in postpartum women was still as high as in trimester 3. Overall, iron storage [mg/kg BW] decreased during pregnancy despite the provision of highly concentrated iron supplements (600 mg ferrous sulphate per day), and women in post partum had a significantly lower iron status and higher proportion of iron deficiency (ID) and iron deficiency anemia (IDA) than women in trimester 1.

Serum zinc during pregnancy decreased concurrently with hematocrit levels from 1st to 2nd trimester was constantly depressed in trimester 3 and rose again in post partum. Serum copper increased as duration of pregnancy progressed (as did cholesterol, triglycerides α-tocopherol) being significantly higher in the following trimester and in each trimesters of gestation when compared to levels in post partum women. By use of suggested lower cut-off values (Hotz, 2003) the prevalence of zinc deficiency was 38% for the women in 1st trimester, about 50% for women in 2nd and 3rd trimester and was highest at 12 weeks post partum with 74% being significantly higher than in trimester 1. Deficient serum levels in copper were rarely detected in pregnant (n=3) and post partum women (n=1). Elevated CRP and AGP confounded SF and copper: SF and serum copper were significantly higher in pregnant and post partum women with elevated levels CRP (>5mg/L) or AGP(>1g/L); however, significant differences between individual groups remained and were still obvious after exclusion of those women with increased CRP or AGP.

Multiple regression analysis on determinants for iron status parameters (**Table 3.6.2a-d**) revealed that hematocrit and age were positive predictors for iron status during pregnancy and in post partum. Gestational age at blood draw (or instead 'weeks of provided iron supplements'), to be Muslim and high body mass index in trimester 1 predicted low serum ferritin and high sTfR and therefore low iron status in pregnancy. Elevated CRP confounded serum ferritin (by mean of its increase) in pregnant women while increased AGP was highly positively associated with serum ferritin but noticeable also with sTfR in post partum.

Table 3.6.1 Iron status, prevalence of IDA, and serum zinc and copper during pregnancy and post partum

Serum	Trimester 1 (5,3 - 12,6)[*] n=118	Trimester 2 (13,0 - 26,6)[*] n=466	Trimester 3 (27,0 - 40,5)[*] n=462	mothers PP week 12 n=89
Ferritin (SF) [1a, 2c] [µg/L]	55.5 (26.9-119)	40.5 (17.5-93.6)	25.8 (11.2-59.8)	41.1 (15.7-108)
SF< 12 µg/L	8% (n=9)	8% (n=35)	20% (n=93)	12% (n=11)
sTfR [mg/L] [1a, 2a]	5.94 (4.30-8.22)	5.95 (4.25-8.33)	7.36 (5.36-10.1)	8.14 (6.15-10.8)
sTfR >8.5 mg/L	13% (n=15)	12% (n=57)	30% (n=140)	36% (n=32)
ID[id] (iron def.) [1a, 2a]	16% (n=19)	17% (n=80)	39% (n=178)	38% (n=34)
Iron storage [1a, 2a] [mg/kg BW]	7.20 (4.03-10.4)	5.58 (2.15-9.0)	3.35 (-0.30-7.0)	4.72 (0.56-8.9)
<0 mg/kg BW [1a, 2c]	7% (n=8)	7% (n=32)	23% (n=106)	16% (n=14)
	N=118	N=464	N=462	N=86
Hematocrit [%] [1a, 2a]	34.7 (3.2)	32.5 (3.4)	32.5 (3.5)	37.4 (3.3)
hct< 30% [1b]	8% (n=9)	18% (n=86)	19% (n=89)	---
IDA[ida1] (& hct<30) [1a]	2% (2)	5% (24)	11% (52)	---
Hemogl. [hb] [g/L] [1a, 2a]	115.5 (10.9)	108.2 (11.2)	108.3 (11.6)	124.7 (10.9)
Anemia [an 1a]	35% (n=41)	35% (n=164)	60% (n=278)	36% (n=31)
IDA[ida2] [1a, 2c (p=0.05)]	7% (8)	9.5% (44)	26% (121)	15% (13)
	n=118	n=466	n=462	n=89
Zinc [mg/L] [1a]	0.638 (0.46-0.88)	0.519 (0.38-0.70)	0.527 (0.39-0.71)	0.601 (0.49-0.74)
% (n) < 0.5-66[* 1c, 2a]	36 (n=43)	49 (n=227)	45 (n=209)	74 (n=66)
Copper [mg/L] [1a, 2a]	1.620 (1.20-2.10)	2.106 (1.64-2.63)	2.268 (1.74-2.87)	1.185 (0.99-1.40)
% (n)< 0.8 [*] mg/L	---	0.4 (n=2)	0.2 (n=1)	1 (n=1)

[**] Figures are mean (SD), geometric mean (2SD range: -/+ 1 SD), and percentage (n)
ID: iron deficiency; IDA: iron deficiency anemia: ID and anemia
[an] anemia: hb<110 g/L in trimester 1 and 3, hb<105 g/L in trimester 2, and hb<120 g/L in post partum
[1] Trimester trend (linear regression), [2] Post partum vs. Trimester 1, [a] $p < 0.001$, [b] $p < 0.01$, [c] $p < 0.05$
[SF] Serum ferritin, [sTfR] sTfR soluble transferrin receptor ; [hb] hemoglobin: hematocrit (hct) x 3.33
[id] ID: iron deficiency defined as SF<12 µg/L or sTfR >8.5 mg/L,
[ida1] ID and hematocrit < 30%; [ida2] ID (SF<12 µg/L or sTfR >8.5 mg/L) and anemia
* zinc cut-offs of <0.56 for T1, <0.50 for T2 and T3, and of <0.66 mg/L for non-pregnant women (Hotz 2003)

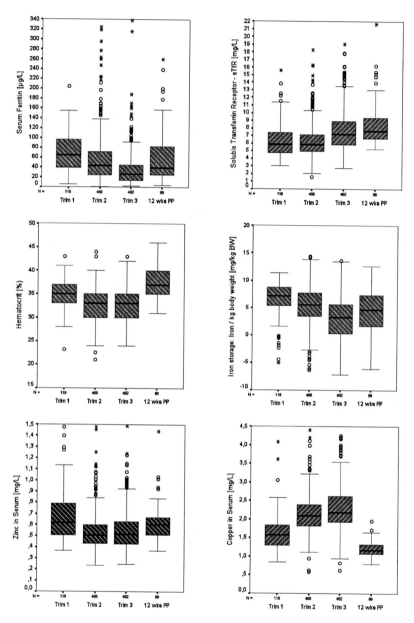

Fig. 3.6.1 Ferritin, sTfR, hematocrit, iron storage, zinc and copper in serum by trimester of pregnancy and at week 12 post partum

Table 3.6.2 Determinants of iron status parameters

a. serum ferritin in pregnancy [log e µg/L], n=1044

	B	S. E.	Beta	t	Sig.	Adj. R^2
(Constant)	3,452	,256		13,49	,000	
EGA at blood draw [weeks][1]	-,031	,003	-,315	-10,92	,000	,106
Muslim (=1)	-,355	,068	-,151	-5,21	,000	,122
CRP >5 mg/L (=1)	,236	,065	,106	3,65	,000	,134
Hematocrit [%]	,027	,007	,106	3,65	,000	,144

b. soluble transferrin receptor (sTfR) in pregnancy [log e mg/L], n=1044

	B	S. E.	Beta	t	Sig.	Adj. R^2
(Constant)	1,163	,249		4,67	,000	
EGA at blood draw [weeks]	,012	,001	,303	10,45	,000	,102
Hematocrit [%]	-,013	,003	-,132	-4,51	,000	,112
BMI, trimester 1 [kg/m^2]	,324	,080	,120	4,06	,000	,122
Age, adm. [years]	-,005	,002	-,107	-3,62	,000	,133
Muslim (=1)	,081	,027	,087	3,03	,003	,140

c. serum ferritin post partum [√ µg/L], n=651

	B	S. E.	Beta	t	Sig.	Adj. R^2
(Constant)	-1,600	1,225		-1,31	,192	
Hematocrit (pp) [%]	,186	,031	,224	6,06	,000	,047
AGP >1 g/L [=1]	1,484	,294	,187	5,05	,000	,079
Age [years]	,066	,015	,169	4,38	,000	,093
Betel nut, daily [=1]	-,840	,240	-,135	-3,50	,001	,109
Post partum group [0,1,2]	-,355	,142	-,093	-2,50	,013	,117

d. soluble transferrin receptor (sTfR) in post partum [log e mg/L], n=658

	B	S. E.	Beta	t	Sig.	Adj. R^2
(Constant)	2,226	,063		35,09	,000	
Post partum group [0,1,2]	-,085	,020	-,165	-4,33	,000	,028
AGP >1 g/L [=1]	,129	,041	,121	3,17	,002	,043
Betel nut, daily [=1]	,122	,033	,146	3,67	,000	,052
Age [years]	-,007	,002	-,133	-3,34	,001	,067

Further betel but consumption showed a negative impact on iron status in post partum. Increasing number of post partum group (PP=0, PP1=1, PP2=2) was associated with lower ferritin but even more important with lower sTfR. Group comparison in pregnant women showed a significant higher sTfR in 2007 (6.7 vs. 6.38 mg/L) despite significantly more weeks of provided iron supplements than in 2004 (13.9 vs. 12.2 weeks). However, post partum group (PP, PP1, PP2) itself was a predictor for sTfR in post partum which was significantly lower in PP1 as well as in PP2 than in PP (**Table 3.6.2-c-d; 3.6.3**) reflecting the improvement of tissue iron status.

Table 3.6.3 Iron status, zinc and copper in post partum

Serum	mothers PP 2004, N=89	mothers PP 1 2004, N=99	mothers PP2 2007, N=470
Ferritin [µg/L]	41.1 (15.7-108)	38.3 (15.0-98.7)	35.0 (14.4-85.3)
SF< 12 µg/L	12% (n=11)	16% (n=16)	12% (n=57)
sTfR [mg/L] [1b, 2a]	8.14 [b, a] (6.15-10.8)	7.27 (5.46-9.7)	6.81 (4.63-10.0)
sTfR >8.5 mg/L [1]	36% (n=32) [c]	21% (n=21)	27% (n=129)
ID[id] (iron def.) [1]	38% (n=34) [d]	26% (n=26)	33% (n=154)
Iron storage	4.72 [-6.2 - 12.6]	5.25 [-6.1 - 12.7]	5.10 [-10.6 - 11.4]
<0 [mg/kg BW] [(yd)]	16% (n=14)	17% (n=17)	11.5% (n=54)
	N=86	N=96	N=469
Hematocrit [%]	37.4 (3.3)	37.3 (2.8)	37.9 (3.4)
Hemogl. [hb] [g/L]	124.7 (10.9)	124.3 (9.4)	126.1 (11.2)
Anemia [an]	36% (n=31)	34% (n=33)	30% (n=140)
IDA[ida]	15% (13)	15% (14)	13% (60)
	N=89	N=99	N=470
Zinc [mg/L] [1c, 2b]	0.601 [c, b]	0.646	0.651
	(0.486-0.744)	(0.514-0.811)	(0.471-0.901)
% (n)< 0.66 mg/L [1, 2]	74 [b] (66)	51 (50)	56 (261)
Copper [mg/L] [2]	1.176 (0.99-1.40)	1.161 (1.00-1.35) [c]	1.211 (0.97-1.50)
breast milk	N=88	N=96	
Iron [mg/L] [1]	0.240 [c] (0.15-0.39)	0.288 (0.15-0.54)	
Iron / milk fat [1]	10.93 [c]	13.18	
[mg/kg]	(7.40-16.1)	(7.22-24.0)	
Zinc [mg/L]	1.775 (1.13-2.57)	1.781 (1.13-2.58)	
Zinc / milk fat	77.25	77.88	
[mg/kg]	(45.3-131.8)	(45.3-134.0)	
Copper [mg/L]	0.279 (0.075)	0.280 (0.066)	
Copper / milk fat	12.16	12.40	
[mg/kg]	(7.3-20.3)	(7.9-19.4)	

[**] Figures are geometric mean (2 SD range: -/+ 1 SD), median [range], mean (SD), and percentage (n)
[1] PP1, [2] PP2 different to respective other (PP) group: [a] $p < 0.001$, [b] $p < 0.01$, [c] $p < 0.05$, [d] $p < 0.1$)
[SF] Serum ferritin, [sTfR] sTfR soluble transferrin receptor; [hb] hemoglobin: hematocrit (hct) x 3.33
[id] ID: iron deficiency defined as SF<12 µg/L or sTfR >8.5 mg/L, [an] anemia: hb<120 g/L in post partum,
[ida] ID (SF<12 µg/L or sTfR >8.5 mg/L) and anemia; [yd] difference between 2007 and 2004: $p < 0.1$

Multiple regression analysis shows that the provision of micronutrient enriched flour (MEF) was a highly positive predictor of serum zinc levels in both pregnancy and in post partum (**Table 3.6.4a-b**). In 2006 zinc levels in each trimester of pregnancy were significantly higher and proportions of women with zinc deficiency were significantly lower than in respective trimesters in 2004 (**Fig. 3.6.2, Table 3.6.5**). Post partum women (PP1, PP2) who were provided with the MEF had significantly higher serum zinc, lower sTfR (indicating improved iron status) and significantly lower proportion of women with zinc deficiency than those women (PP) who were not (**Table 3.6.3**). The higher serum zinc in PP1 was not associated with an increase of respective zinc levels in milk. But the improvement in iron status by means of lower sTfR and therefore improvement of 'tissue iron' in PP1 was simultaneously associated with a significantly higher milk iron (per volume and per milk fat) than in the PP group.

Table 3.6.4 Determinants of zinc in serum of pregnant and post partum women

a. serum zinc in pregnancy [log e mg/L], n=1046

	B	S. E.	Beta	t	Sig.	Adj. R^2
(Constant)	-,759	,041		-18,644	,000	
2006 (prov. MEF=1) vs. 2004 (no MEF=0)	,201	,018	,325	11,173	,000	**,097**
Trimester (1, 2,3)	-,076	,014	-,165	-5,571	,000	,118
sTfR > 8.5 =1	,059	,023	,076	2,577	,010	,123

b. serum zinc in post partum [log e mg/L], n=650

	B	S. E.	Beta	t	Sig.	Adj. R^2
(Constant)	-,982	,146		-6,720	,000	
Hematocrit (pp) [%]	,015	,004	,163	4,127	,000	,037
Flour (MEF) provided=1	,088	,034	,099	2,601	,010	**,044**
Smoking [yes=1]	,084	,027	,125	3,074	,002	,050
Ferritin (pp) < 12 µg/L =1	-,085	,035	-,095	-2,407	,016	,055
Age [years] at admission	-,004	,002	-,092	-2,250	,025	,061

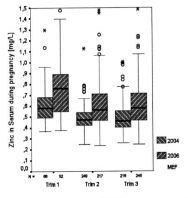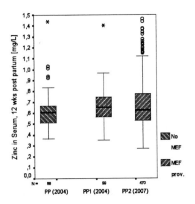

Fig. 3.6.2 Impact by MEF on serum zinc during pregnancy and in post partum

Table 3.6.5 Impact by MEF on serum zinc levels and prevalence of zinc deficiency during pregnancy

2004 vs. 2006 -MEF	Trimester 1		Trimester 2		Trimester 3	
	2004	2006	2004	2006	2004	2006
Zinc [mg/L] [a,b]	0.586	0.710 [b]	0.473	0.577 [a]	0.474	0.578 [a]
% (n) < 0.56, 0.5 mg/L	44	27	64	31 [a]	62	30 [a]
	(n=29/66)	(n=14/52)	(n=159/249)	(n=68(217)	(n=133/216)	(n=76/246)

Mean zinc levels in breast milk were quite high despite low serum zinc levels at 12 weeks post partum. Zinc, copper and in particular iron in milk was highly predicted by the concentration of milk fat in the sample (**Table 3.6.6**). Increasing sTfR and therefore tissue iron deficiency reduced milk iron. Higher serum zinc was even inversely correlated with milk zinc levels, and serum copper didn't show any significant relation to copper values in breast milk.

Table 3.6.6 Predictors of iron, zinc and copper in breast milk

a. iron in breast milk [log e mg/L], n=183

	B	S. E.	Beta	t	Sig.	Adj R^2
(Constant)	-,878	,266		-3,30	,001	
Milk fat [g/L]	,028	,004	,478	7,61	,000	,212
sTfR [log e mg/L]	-,549	,124	-,278	-4,42	,000	,286

b. zinc in breast milk [√ mg/L], n=183

	B	S. E.	Beta	t	Sig.	Adj R^2
(Constant)	1,389	,111		12,52	,000	
Milk fat [g/L]	,007	,002	,269	3,88	,000	,067
Age [years]	-,015	,004	-,357	-3,60	,000	,099
Parity [N babies born]	,033	,014	,233	2,34	,020	,119
Serum zinc pp [ln mg/L]	-,179	,084	-,147	-2,13	,034	,136

c. copper in milk [mg/L]

	B	S. E.	Beta	t	Sig.	Adj R^2
(Constant)	,301	,025		12,29	,000	
Betel nut, daily [=1]	-,039	,013	-,223	-3,09	,002	,072
Milk fat [g/L]	,001	,000	,191	2,74	,007	,109
Age [years]	-,002	,001	-,165	-2,28	,024	,129

Logistic regression analysis revealed that a high hematocrit and younger age decreased the risk for negative iron storage in pregnant and breast-feeding women (**Table 3.6.7**). Gestational age and to be Muslim were risk factors in pregnancy whereas betel nut consumption and smoking increased the risk for negative iron storage in the post partum women. SF, sTfR and iron status in post partum were significantly positively associated with respective iron parameters in pregnancy: women with iron deficiency in pregnancy indicated by 'negative iron storages' were at high risk (5 fold higher risk compared to women with positive iron stores during pregnancy) to be iron deficient in the post partum period.

Table 3.6.7 Risk factors for negative iron storage [mg iron / kg BW < 0]

a. Logistic regression: negative iron storage in pregnancy: N=146/1044 (14%)

	B	S. E.	Wald	Sig.	Exp(B)	95% C.I.	
Constant	1,774	1,069	2,76	,097	5,89		
EGA [weeks]	,089	,013	46,44	,000	1,09	1,07	1,12
Hematocrit, preg [%]	-,163	,029	31,89	,000	,85	,80	,90
Muslim (=1)	,925	,230	16,13	,000	2,52	1,61	3,96
CRP >5 mg/L (=1)	-,675	,285	5,60	,018	,51	,29	,89
Age [years]	-,033	,015	5,08	,024	,97	,94	1,00

b. Logistic regression: negative iron storage in post partum: N=85/650 (13%)

	B	S. E.	Wald	Sig.	Exp(B)	95% C.I.	
Constant	8,236	1,510	29,75	,000	3775,0		
Hematocrit (pp) [%]	-,236	,039	36,23	,000	,79	,73	,85
Betel nut, daily [=1]	,783	,287	7,44	,006	2,19	1,25	3,84
Age [years]	-,073	,022	11,27	,001	,93	,89	,97
Smoking [=1]	,720	,294	5,99	,014	2,05	1,15	3,65

c. follow-up women: negative iron storage (festo<0) in post partum: N=71/565 (13%)

	B	S. E.	Wald	Sig.	Exp(B)	95% C.I.	
Constant	6,617	1,651	16,06	,000	747,9		
Festo in preg < 0*	1,640	,299	30,02	,000	**5,15**	2,87	9,26
Hematocrit (pp) [%]	-,211	,043	23,86	,000	,81	,74	,88
Betel nut, daily [=1]	1,202	,313	14,72	,000	3,33	1,80	6,15
Age [years]	-,060	,024	6,54	,011	,94	,90	,99

* Festo in preg < 0: negative iron storage (mg iron per kg BW <0) in pregnancy

Overall, prevalence of iron and zinc deficiency was high in pregnant and breast-feeding women. Serum zinc in pregnancy and both zinc levels and iron status in post partum increased significantly after the introduction of the micronutrient enriched flour in June 2004. Improved iron status was simultaneously associated with significantly higher iron in breast milk.

3.7 DDT residues in serum and breast milk

DDT residues in serum and breast milk per volume and expressed on a per fat basis in pregnant and post partum women are given in **table 3.7.1, 3.7.2** and **Fig 3.7.1**. The predominant metabolite p,p'-DDE was detected in all serum and breast milk samples. Total DDT in serum ranged between 0.2 and 233 µg/L and in breast milk between 1.8 and 1908 µg/L. DDT compounds correlated highly with each other and with corresponding fat concentrations (cholesterol, triglycerides) in serum and breast milk (**Table 3.7.3, 3.7.4b**).

Table 3.7.1 Serum DDT residues during pregnancy and in post partum

Serum	Trimester 1 n=119	Trimester 2 n=466	Trimester 3 n=462	12 weeks PP n=89
p,p'-DDE [1a, 2b] [µg/L]	6.33 (1.73-23.1)	8.18 (2.06-32.5)	10.34 (2.73-39.1)	10.02 (3.45-29.1)
p,p'-DDD [µg/L]	0.65 (58) (0.22-1.91)	0.75 (265) (0.24-2.35)	0.81 (294) (0.27-2.38)	0.69 (36) (0.22-2.21)
p,p'-DDT [1a, 2a] [µg/L]	2.13 (112) (0.66-6.91)	2.63 (0.69-10.0)	3.23 (0.82-12.7)	3.94 (1.54-10.1)
DDE /DDT [1c, 2b]	3.37 (1.46-7.79)	3.44 (1.52-7.78)	3.34 (1.5-7.42)	2.54 (1.44-4.49)
Total DDT [1a, 2b] [µg/L]	8.73 (2.24-31.0) [0.36-121.2]	11.29 (2.9-43.9) [0.26-213.7]	14.49 (3.89-53.9) [0.22-233.3]	14.72 (5.45-39.7) [1.8-119.4]
Fat [g/L] [1a, 2b] (total serum fat)	5.01 (4.20-5.97)	6.54 (5.37-7.98)	8.43 (6.93-10.3)	5.47 (4.51-6.63)
Total DDT / fat [2b] [mg/kg]	1.723 (0.49-6.08) [0.08-26.2]	1.725 (0.44-6.73) [0.04-35.6]	1.729 (0.47-6.32) [0.03-29.5]	2.693 (0.98-7.40) [0.31-26.53]

** Figures are geometric mean (2SD range: -/+ 1 SD) and range [min-max]
[1] Trimester trend (linear regression), [a] $p < 0.001$, [b] $p < 0.01$, [c] $p < 0.05$
[2] Post partum women in 2004 (n=89) different to trimester 1 in 2004-2006: [a] $p < 0.001$, [b] $p < 0.01$
Total DDT: sum of p,p'-DDE, p,p'-DDD, o,p'-DDT, and p,p'-DDT.
Fat (total serum fat): sum of cholesterol, triglycerides and estimated phospholipids

The positive associations with serum fat explained partly the significant increase of DDT residues with gestational age. Once adjusted for total serum fat, mean total DDT residues didn't differ between trimesters of pregnancy. DDT residues in the initially post partum group in 2004 (n=89) were significantly higher than respective mean values of 1st trimester women of 2004 and 2006.

Table 3.7.2 DDT residues in post partum: levels in serum and breast milk

Serum	mothers PP n=89	mothers PP1 n=99	mothers PP2 n=470
p,p'-DDE [2] [µg/L]	10.02 [a] (3.45-29.1)	7.70 [a] (2.03-29.2)	4.78 (1.44-15.8)
p,p'-DDD [µg/L]	0.69 (36) (0.22-2.21)	0.65 (43) (0.22-1.91)	0.56 (479) (0.30-1.05)
p,p'-DDT [2] [µg/L]	3.94 [a] (1.54-10.1)	2.96 [a] (0.92-9.48)	1.56 (0.77-3.16)
ppDDE / ppDDT [2] [µg/L / µg/L]	2.54 [b] (1.44-4.49)	2.78 (1.64-4.72)	3.06 (1.44-6.50)
Total DDT [2] [µg/L]	14.72 [a] (5.45-39.7) [1.8-119.4]	10.8 [b] (2.92-39.9) [0.3-88.3]	7.34 (2.72-19.8) [0.9-101.8]
Fat [g/L] (total serum fat)	5.47 (4.51-6.63)	5.62 (4.62-6.84)	5.61 (4.59-6.85)
Total DDT / fat [2] [mg/kg] [(PP1vs.PP:c)]	2.693 [a] (0.98-7.40) [0.31-26.53]	1.920 [b] (0.53-6.98) [0.06-17.37]	1.310 (0.48-3.60) [0.15-19.9]
Breast Milk	**N=88**	**N=96**	**N=464**
p,p'-DDE [2] [µg/L]	90.0 [a] (28.5-284)	77.8 [a] (21.2-286)	41.8 (9.2-189)
p,p'-DDD [2] [µg/L]	4.19 [a] (86) (1.25-14.0)	4.33 [a] (91) (1.10-17.1)	0.77 (53) (0.24-2.48)
p,p'-DDT [2] [µg/L]	37.3 [a] (11.6-120)	32.9 [a] (94) (8.82-123)	11.8 (4.16-33.6)
ppDDE / ppDDT [2] [µg/L / µg/L]	2.41 [a] (1.38-4.24)	2.54 [a] (1.59-4.05)	3.53 (1.70-7.33)
Total DDT [2] [µg/L]	136.6 (43.9-425) [2.7-1908]	114.5 (30.0-437) [1.8-1809]	56.5 (14.0-228) [2.9-1277]
Fat in milk [g/L] [2] (triglycerides)	22.7 [a] (13.5-34.3)	20.5 [a] (12.6-30.3)	28.9 (17.8-42.8)
Total DDT / fat [2] [mg/kg]	6.36 [a] (2.27-17.8) [0.54-59.33]	5.87 [a] (1.72-20.0) [0.22-48.13]	2.05 (0.52-8.08) [0.10-47.6]

[**] Figures are geometric mean (2SD range: -/+ 1 SD) and range [min-max]
[2] PP2 different to PP1 and PP: [a] $p < 0.001$, [b] $p < 0.01$, [c] $p < 0.05$
Total DDT: sum of p,p'-DDE, p,p'-DDD, o,p'-DDT, and p,p'-DDT.
Fat (in serum): sum of cholesterol, triglycerides and estimated phospholipids. Fat in milk: triglycerides

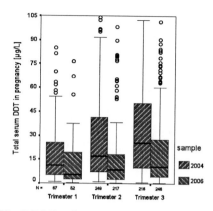 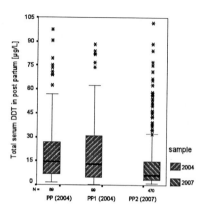

Fig. 3.7.1 Total serum DDT residues by trimester, year and post partum group

Total serum DDT residues in pregnant and post partum women were predominantly explained by the years of residence in Thailand, parity and the year of sample collection (**Table 3.7.3**). Total years of residence in Thailand were highly and positively associated with DDT residues whereas a higher number of born children (parity) and therefore possible number of former breast-fed infants was a predictor for lower serum DDT (**Fig. 3.7.2**).

Table 3.7.3 Predictors of total DDT residues

a. Total DDT in serum during pregnancy [$\log_e$ µg/L], n=1044

	B	S. E.	Beta	T	Sig.	Adj R^2
(Constant)	1,247	,243		5,1	,000	
Years in Thailand	,098	,005	,471	20,6	,000	,221
Parity (born babies)	-,240	,016	-,346	-15,0	,000	,330
Year 2007 (1) vs. 2004 (0)	-,845	,062	-,315	-13,7	,000	,406
Cholesterol s1 [mmol/L])	,148	,027	,143	5,5	,000	,444
Weight, trimester 1 [kg]	,019	,004	,102	4,4	,000	,454
Triglycerides [mmol/L]	,129	,030	,113	4,3	,000	,463

b. Total serum DDT residues in post partum [$\log_e$ µg/L], n=658

	B	S. E.	Beta	T	Sig.	Adj. R^2
(Constant)	1,419	,285		4,9	,000	
Years in Thailand	,075	,005	,456	14,7	,000	,201
Parity (born babies)	-,200	,017	-,369	-11,8	,000	,310
Year 2007 (1) vs. 2004 (0)	-,552	,073	-,232	-7,6	,000	,363
Weight, 12 weeks pp [kg]	,016	,005	,109	3,5	,001	,377
Cholesterol s2 [mmol/L]	,106	,034	,099	3,2	,002	,385

Samples collected in 2007 had significant lower mean DDT than those collected in 2004, and mother's weight and serum fat were positively associated with DDT residues. Serum DDT in the post partum period correlated highly and positively to respective serum DDT in pregnancy as well as to the several fold higher DDT residues in breast milk (**Fig. 3.7.3; 3.7.4**). Fat adjusted total DDT in pregnancy explained 85% of the variation in fat adjusted total DDT in post partum, which by itself explained >80% of the variation in total DDT and fat adjusted total DDT in breast milk (**Table 3.7.4**).

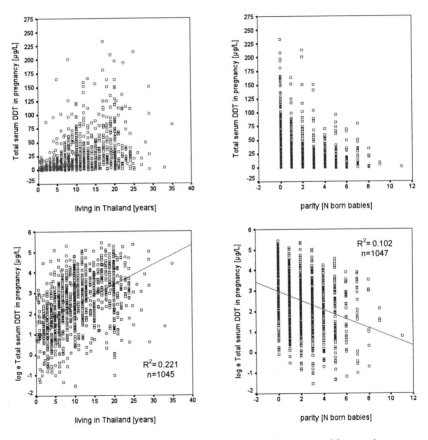

Fig. 3.7.2 Impact by years of staying in Thailand and number of former born babies on total serum DDT residues in pregnancy

Table 3.7.4 Determinants of DDT residues (serum and milk) in post partum

a. Fat adjusted total serum DDT in post partum [$\log_e$ µg/g], n=569 (follow-up)

	B	S.E.	Beta	T	Sig.	Adj. R^2
(Constant)	,136	,019		7,293	,000	
Total DDT per serum fat in pregnancy [(log e) µg/g]	,727	,014	,914	53,503	,000	**,834**

b. Total DDT in breast milk [log e µg/L], n=643

	B	S.E.	Beta	T	Sig.	Adj. R^2
(Constant)	2,919	,110		26,6	,000	
Total DDT per serum fat PP [(log e) µg/g]	1,137	,019	,882	58,9	,000	**,805**
Fat in milk [($\sqrt{}$) g/L]	,293	,018	,247	16,2	,000	,850
sample 2004 (1) 2007 (2)	-,391	,048	-,126	-8,1	,000	,863

c. Total DDT per milk fat [log e µg/gram], n=643

	B	S. E.	Beta	T	Sig.	Adj. R^2
(Constant)	1,348	,085		15,9	,000	
Total DDT per serum fat in post partum [log e µg/g]	1,132	,019	,881	58,4	,000	**,839**
sample 2004 (1) 2007 (2)	-,474	,047	-,153	-10,2	,000	,861

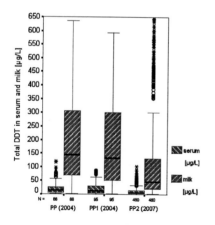 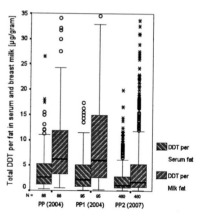

Fig 3.7.3 Total DDT in serum and breast milk by post partum groups

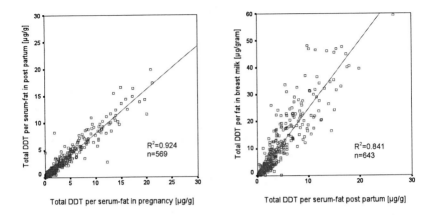

Fig. 3.7.4 Relation between serum fat adjusted DDT residues in pregnancy and post partum and between fat adjusted DDT in serum and breast milk

The DDT-induced increase of plasma retinol as previously described in pregnant Karen from Maela was no longer obviously in the present study. α-Tocopherol showed significantly positive associations to DDT residues in both pregnant and post partum women (Pearson 0.228, 0.121, $p < 0.001$ for total DDT); the positive correlations were still significant after both DDT and α-tocopherol were adjusted for serum fat (Pearson 0.149, 0.146, $p < 0.001$). Nevertheless, the positive associations between DDT residues and α-tocopherol are most likely due to their strong correlation to serum fat.

3.8 Pregnancy outcomes: birth weights and infants anthropometry

Pregnancy outcomes are summarized in **Table 3.8.1**. In 2004 mean birth weight and newborns anthropometry didn't differ between the PP and PW1 group. In 2006/7 mean birth weight, gestational age at outcome and newborns length, arm- and head circumference improved significantly and proportion of low birth weight and of intrauterine growth retardation (IUGR) were significantly lower than in 2004.

Table 3.8.1 Pregnancy outcomes: birth weights and infants anthropometry [a]

Pregnancy outcomes	PP (2004) N= 89	PW1 (2004) N= 533	PW2 (2006/07) N= 515
Lost / left camp [n]	1 (BW)	4	5
Abortions [n]		6	10
Stillbirth [n]		3 (1 BW < 1000)	3 (2 BWs)
Twins [n]		8	4
BW day ≥4 or ? [n]	1	11	6
	N= 87	**N= 501**	**N= 489**
Birth weight [2]	2982 (405)	2945 (449) [b]	3047 (459)
	2951 (442) [a]		
EGA at outcome [2]	38.7 (1.1) [a]	38.9 (1.6) [b]	39.2 (1.6)
	38.8 (1.5) [a]		
Preterm [%, (n)]	3.5 (n=3)	7.6 (n=38)	5.9 (n=29)
Sex, male [%]	55	52	54
LBW [N (%)] [2] (< 2500g)	12.6 (n=11)	14.5 (n=73) [b]	9.2 (n=45)
	14.1% (n=83/588) [c]		
IUGR [% (N)] [2] (<2500g, EGA ≥37)	11.9 (n=10/84)	10.6 (n=49/463) [c]	6.3 (n=29/460)
	10.8 (n=59/547) [c]		
	N= 61	**N= 412**	**N= 484**
Length [cm] [2]	49.2 (2.1)	48.7 (2.2) [b]	49.1 (2.1)
	48.8 (2.2) [c]		
Sex, male [%]	51	52	53
Arm - [cm] [2] circumference	9.9 (1.2) [a]	10.1 (1.4) [a]	10.6 (1.0)
	10.1 (1.3) [a]		
Head - [cm] [2] circumference	31.9 (1.5) [c]	32.0 (1.5) [a]	32.4 (1.4)
	32.0 (1.5) [a]		

[a] figures are means (SD) for birth weight, length, arm- and head circumference
[2] PW2 different to respective other groups (PW1, PP - 2004): [a] $p < 0.001$, [b] $p < 0.01$, [c] $p < 0.05$
* N=411 for arm and head circumference in PW1 group

64

The predominant predictor accounting for between 16 and 30% of the variability (R^2) in newborns' weight and anthropometry was gestational age at delivery, followed by mother's weight, height and parity (**Fig. 3.8.1**, **Table 3.8.2, and 3.8.3**).

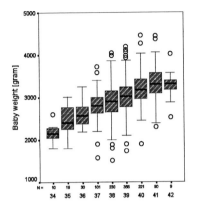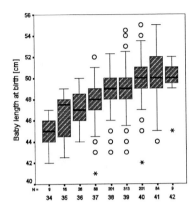

Fig. 3.8.1 Babies weight and length at birth by gestational week

Table 3.8.2 Multivariate linear regression on birth weight [grams]

a. mothers 1st trimester weight included in the model: n=1078, adj. R^2= 39.5%

	B	S. E	Beta	t	Sig.	Adj R^2
(Constant)	-4276,4	400,8		-10,67	,000	
EGA at outcome [weeks]	143,1	7,03	,495	20,35	,000	,298
Mothers weight trim. 1 [kg]	13,8	1,7	,221	7,98	,000	,369
Height at admission [cm]	7,5	2,3	,088	3,27	,001	,374
Parity (babies born) [N]	44,4	8,5	,184	5,25	,000	,378
Age at admission [years]	-7,7	2,4	-,113	-3,18	,002	,386
Smoking yes/no [yes=1]	-83,2	26,3	-,081	-3,17	,002	,391
Baby sex [male=1]	64,3	21,8	,070	2,95	,003	**,395**

b. mothers 1st trimester weight excluded from the model: n=1078, adj. R^2= 36%

	B	S. E	Beta	t	Sig.	Adj R^2
(Constant)	-5088,7	399,4		-12,74	,000	
EGA at outcome [weeks]	145,0	7,3	,501	20,00	,000	,298
Height at admission [cm]	15,9	2,1	,187	7,58	,000	,333
Parity (babies born) [N]	46,4	8,7	,192	5,33	,000	,342
Smoking yes/no [yes=1]	-115,0	26,7	-,112	-4,32	,000	,353
Baby sex [male=1]	61,9	22,4	,068	2,77	,006	,358
2004 (=1), 2007 (=2)	47,6	22,5	,052	2,11	,035	,360
Age at admission [years]	-5,2	2,5	-,075	-2,09	,037	**,362**

Male infant was a positive while smoking was a significant negative predictor for infant's weight and length at birth. Mother's age was negatively associated with BW if both parity and age were included in the models.

Table 3.8.3 Linear regression on newborns anthropometry

a. Infant's lengths at birth (n=957), adjusted R^2 = 32.3%

	B	S. E.	Beta	t	Sig.	Adj R^2
(Constant)	14,98	2,19		6,85	,000	
EGA at outcome [weeks]	,615	,039	,436	15,91	,000	,236
Mothers 1st trim. weight [kg]	,048	,009	,159	5,13	,000	,287
Baby sex [male=1]	,610	,117	,140	5,22	,000	,305
Height at admission [cm]	,048	,012	,119	3,92	,000	,314
Smoking yes/no [yes=1]	-,496	,139	-,102	-3,56	,000	,320
Parity (babies born) [N]	,080	,033	,069	2,41	,016	,323

b. Infant's arm circumference (n= 956), adjusted R^2 = 24%

	B	S. E.	Beta	t	Sig.	Adj R^2
(Constant)	-2,302	,898		-2,56	,010	
EGA at outcome [weeks]	,271	,023	,342	11,74	,000	,164
Mothers 1st trim. weight [kg]	,028	,005	,166	5,71	,000	,201
Group 2004 (=1), 2006/07 (=2)	,417	,070	,170	5,98	,000	,229
Parity (babies born) [N]	,077	,020	,119	3,91	,000	,237
Smoking yes/no [yes=1]	-,188	,083	-,069	-2,26	,024	,240

c. Infants head circumference (n=956), adj. R^2 = 26.6%

	B	S. E	Beta	t	Sig.	Adj R^2
(Constant)	12,48	1,55		8,06	,000	
EGA at outcome [weeks]	,368	,027	,381	13,40	,000	,191
Mothers 1st trim. weight [kg]	,029	,007	,144	4,47	,000	,229
Parity (babies born) [N]	,133	,022	,169	5,99	,000	,254
Group 2004 (=1), 2006/07 (=2)	,232	,083	,078	2,78	,006	,259
Height at admission [cm]	,021	,009	,076	2,40	,017	,263
Baby sex [male=1]	,196	,083	,066	2,37	,018	,266

Infants born in 2006/07 were associated with significantly higher weight and arm- and head circumference than those born in 2004. The significant higher birth weight in 2007 was most likely due to significantly higher maternal weight (**see Table 3.1.1**) and increase in gestational age (**see Table 3.8.1**): year of birth (2004 =1 vs. 2007=2) appeared in the model after exclusion of mother's 1st trimester weight (**Table 3.8.2b**). Multivariate logistic regression revealed that gestational age, 1st trimester weight, nulliparity, smoking and female gender of the newborn were the main risk factors for low birth weight (LBW), intra-uterine growth retardation (IUGR), small for gestional age (SGA) (**Table 3.8.4 a-c**). Higher gestational age and mother's 1st trimester weight decreased whereas smoking, nulliparity and female gender of the newborn increased the risk of LBW, IUGR, and SGA. Nulliparity (first born child) and low mothers weight were significant risk factors for preterm birth (**Table 3.8.4d**)

Table 3.8.4 Predictors and risk factors of low birth weight (LBW), small for gestational age birth (SGA) and intrauterine growth retardation (IUGR)

a. Predictors of LBW (<2500 gram), n=129/1076 (12%)

	B	S. E.	Wald	Sig.	Exp(B)	95,0% C.I.	
Constant	29,851	3,065	94,828	,000	9,2 E+12		
EGA at outcome [weeks]	-,716	,075	90,943	,000	,49	,42	,57
Mothers weight, Trim. 1 [kg]	-,109	,021	28,103	,000	,90	,86	,93
Smoking yes/no [yes=1]	,705	,240	8,663	,003	2,03	1,27	3,24
Nulliparous [yes=1]	,670	,254	6,980	,008	1,95	1,19	3,21
Baby sex [female=1]	,488	,222	4,836	,028	1,63	1,05	2,52

b. Predictors of IUGR (LBW at term): n= 88/1005 (9%)

	B	S.E.	Wald	Sig.	Exp(B)	95,0% C.I.	
Constant	27,328	4,873	31,447	,000	7,4 E +11		
EGA at outcome [weeks]	-,647	,123	27,86	,000	,52	,41	,67
Mothers weight, Trim. 1 [kg]	-,115	,023	25,18	,000	,89	,85	,93
Smoking [yes=1]	,866	,258	11,28	,001	2,38	1,43	3,94
Nulliparous [yes=1]	,766	,281	7,42	,006	2,15	1,24	3,74
Baby sex [female=1]	,624	,240	6,75	,009	1,87	1,17	2,99

c. Predictors of SGA birth (10th percentile per EGA 34-41/42), n= 105/1064 (10%)

	B	S.E.	Wald	Sig.	Exp(B)	95,0% C.I.	
Constant	1,907	,913	4,37	,037	6,73		
Mothers weight, Trim. 1 [kg]	-,094	,020	22,90	,000	,91	,88	,95
Nulliparous [yes=1]	1,087	,242	20,14	,000	2,96	1,84	4,77
Smoking [yes=1]	,830	,237	12,23	,000	2,29	1,44	3,65
Baby sex [female=1]	,763	,218	12,19	,000	2,14	1,40	3,29

d. Predictors of preterm birth (< 37 weeks EGA), n= 71/1076 (7%)

	B	S.E.	Wald	Sig.	Exp(B)	95,0% C.I.	
Constant	-,235	,985	,057	,811	,79		
Nulliparous [yes=1]	1,005	,253	15,83	,000	2,73	1,67	4,48
Mothers weight, Trim. 1 [kg]	-,059	,021	7,60	,006	,94	,91	,98

Logistic regression on LBW regarding both valid birth weights and corresponding maternal blood micronutrient levels (PP1, PP2) revealed that lowest quintile of gestational age (≤38.1 week) and of mother's 1st trimester weight (≤ 42 kg) compared to respective highest quintiles (≥40.2 weeks and ≥53 kg) increased the risk for LBW babies (< 2500 grams) by > 13.5 and 6 fold respectively (**Table 3.8.5**); in addition nulliparity (parity=0) and smoking status were identified as risk factors of LBW.

3.8.5 Logistic regression on low birth weight: <2500 grams, n=118/ 989 (12%)

	B	Wald	Sig.	Exp(B)	95 % C.I.	
Constant	-2,629	209,02	,000	,072		
EGA ≥ 40.2 [weeks]		**69,39**	,000	control		
EGA in 4th quintile (39.4-40.1)	-,712	,92	,339	,49	,11	2,11
EGA in 3rd quintile (39-39.3)	,915	3.00	,083	2,50	,89	7,04
EGA in 2nd quintile (38.2-38.6)	1,619	10,27	,001	**5,05**	1,87	13,59
EGA in lowest quintile (< 38.1)	2,605	28,49	,000	**13,53**	5,20	35,23
Mothers weight ≥ 53 [kg]		**27,10**	,000	control		
Weight in 4th quintile (49-52.9)	,881	3,67	,056	2,41	,98	5,94
Weight in 3rd quintile (45-48.9)	,811	3,26	,071	2,25	,93	5,43
Weight in 2nd quintile (42-44.9)	,641	1,97	,160	1,90	,78	4,64
Weight in lowest quintile ≤ 42	1,790	18,04	,000	**5,99**	2,62	13,69
Parity N ≥ 5		**12,42**	,014	control		
Parity N=3-4	-,071	,03	,866	,93	,41	2,13
Parity N=2	-,442	,93	,336	,64	,26	1,58
Parity N=1	,195	,22	,637	1,22	,54	2,73
Parity N=0 (Nulliparous)	,753	3,47	,063	**2,12**	,96	4,70
Smoking [yes=1]	,739	**8,66**	,003	**2,09**	1,28	3,42

3.9 Impact by DDT and micronutrients on pregnancy outcomes

Univariate analysis on birth weight revealed a significant impact by either continuous or categorized (quintiles) serum DDT in pregnancy. Mean birth weight in the highest quintile was significantly lower than in each of the lower quintiles of DDT residues. But neither highest DDT category nor continuous serum DDT had a significant effect on the risk of low birth weight (LBW<2500 grams), intra-uterine growth retardation (IUGR) or small for gestational age (SGA) newborns. Smoking, nulliparity and female gender of the newborn but not DDT increased the risk of LBW, IUGR, SGA and preterm birth. However, the crude inverse association between continuous serum fat adjusted maternal total DDT [µg/g fat] and newborn birth weight remained significant in multivariate regression analysis adjusted for gestational age, mothers 1st trimester weight, height and age, infant's sex and smoking status (**Table 3.9.1**). Overall the model explained 40% (adj. R^2) of which EGA at delivery alone accounted for 30% of the variability of infant's birth weight. DDT was a significant negative predictor but had a small effect on birth weight compared to parity, smoking or infant's sex.

Table 3.9.1 Association between maternal serum DDT [µg/g fat] during pregnancy and birth weight (BW) [grams], n=1076

a. crude association	B	S.E.	95% CI		T	Sig.
Constant	3026,9	17,44	2992,6	3061,1	173,58	,000
Total DDT per serum fat in pregnancy [µg/g]	-9,12	2,79	-14,60	-3,64	-3,27	,001

b. adjusted association	B	S. E	Beta	T	Sig.	Adj. R^2
(Constant)	-4249,98	397,85		-10,68	,000	
EGA at date of outcome	142,23	7,03	,492	20,25	,000	,300
Mothers weight, Trim. 1 [kg]	13,98	1,73	,223	8,08	,000	,370
Height at admission [cm]	7,64	2,26	,090	3,38	,001	,376
Parity (babies born) [N]	40,92	8,66	,169	4,73	,000	,380
Age at admission [years]	-7,76	2,42	-,113	-3,20	,001	,388
Smoking [yes=1]	-87,11	26,24	-,085	-3,32	,001	,393
Baby sex [male=1]	62,76	21,73	,069	2,89	,004	,397
Total DDT per serum fat in pregnancy [µg/g]	-4,78	2,30	-,052	-2,08	,038	,399

Similar to birth weight, maternal DDT was still a significant predictor of gestational age at outcome (EGA) or length of gestation in multivariate regression analysis but explained much less in variance than did the covariates mothers' weight, parity and smoking (**Table 3.9.2**).

Table 3.9.2 Association between maternal serum DDT [µg/g fat] during pregnancy and length of gestation [weeks], n=1076

a. crude association	B	S.E.	95% CI		T	Sig.
Constant	39,09	,060	38,97	39,21	647,24	,000
Total DDT per serum fat in pregnancy [µg/g]	-,025	,010	-,044	-,006	-2,60	,009

b. adjusted association	B	S.E.	Beta	T	Sig.	Adj. R^2
(Constant)	37,721	,322		117,03	,000	
Mothers weight trim. 1 [kg]	,026	,007	,121	3,96	,000	,020
Parity (babies born) [N]	,093	,028	,111	3,33	,001	,029
Smoking [yes=1]	-,371	,113	-,105	-3,29	,001	,037
Total DDT per serum fat in pregnancy [µg/g]	-,021	,010	-,065	-2,05	,040	**,040**

c. adjusted association	B	S.E.	Beta	T	Sig.	Adj. R^2
(Constant)	34,820	1,363		25,55	,000	
Mothers weight trim. 1 [kg]	,019	,007	,087	2,52	,012	,020
Parity (babies born) [N]	,095	,028	,114	3,43	,001	,029
Smoking [yes=1]	-,374	,113	-,106	-3,32	,001	,037
Height at admission [cm]	,022	,010	,074	2,19	,029	,041
Total DDT per serum fat in pregnancy [µg/g]	-,020	,010	-,063	-1,20	**,046**	**,043**

Univariate analysis on birth weight and circulating micronutrients or DDT during pregnancy indicated positive associations to crude, gestational age (EGA) and serum fat adjusted α-tocopherol and negative associations to EGA adjusted ferritin, iron stores, and retinol, fat adjusted DDT as well as to elevated AGP (>1g/L) and high hematocrit levels (≥37.5%). Multivariate regression on birth weight revealed significant positive relations to fat adjusted α-tocopherol and negative associations with EGA adjusted iron stores and fat adjusted DDT (**Table 3.9.3**).

Table 3.9.3 Relation between maternal circulating serum micronutrients and DDT during pregnancy and birth weight

	B	S. E.	Beta	T	Sig.
(Constant)	2834,76	97,90		28,96	,000
Group 2004 (=1), 2006/07 (=2)	76,09	30,05	,082	2,53	,012
Iron storage [mg/kg BW], adj. [1]	-13,00	4,18	-,098	-3,11	,002
Total DDT / fat [µg/g]	-8,83	3,16	-,091	-2,79	,005
α-tocopherol / fat [µmol/g]	58,86	25,96	,072	2,27	,024

[1] iron storage adjusted = (iron storage) + (0.161*EGA at blood draw)

70

α-Tocopherol was positively while DDT and iron stores were still significantly inversely associated with birth weight in multivariate model including predominantly predictors of pregnancy outcomes (**Table 3.9.4 a**). In addition highest hematocrits (≥37.5%) during pregnancy were negatively associated with newborns weight. Further elevated AGP had a marginal significant negative effect (B= -138.45 grams (SE 73.30), p=0.059) on birth weight (data not shown). Thiamine di-phosphate (TDP) per volume and per hemoglobin, both un-adjusted and adjusted for EGA, were significant positive predictors of babies' lengths (**Table 3.9.4 b**).

Table 3.9.4 Impact by micronutrients and DDT on pregnancy outcomes

a. Multiple regression on birth weight [grams], n=988, R^2= 41.4%

	B	S. E.	Beta	T	Sig.	Adj R^2
(Constant)	-4492,58	416,55		-10,79	,000	
EGA at date of outcome	142,96	7,14	,500	20,02	,000	,313
Mothers weight trim. 1 [kg]	12,20	1,79	,192	6,83	,000	,378
Height at admission [cm])	8,23	2,36	,096	3,49	,001	,385
Iron storage [mg/kg BW], adj.[1]	**-10,13**	**3,26**	**-,076**	**-3,11**	**,002**	**,391**
Parity [N babies born]	23,00	6,67	,094	3,45	,001	,396
Smoking [yes=1]	-94,70	27,37	-,091	-3,46	,001	,402
Baby sex [male=1]	66,77	22,63	,072	2,95	,003	,406
Hematocrit ≥ 37.5% [yes=1]	**-109,69**	**41,68**	**-,064**	**-2,63**	**,009**	**,410**
Total DDT / fat [µg/g]	**-5,45**	**2,51**	**-,056**	**-2,17**	**,030**	**,412**
α-tocopherol / fat [µmol/g]	**42,39**	**20,40**	**,052**	**2,08**	**,038**	**,414**

[1] iron storage adjusted for gestational age (EGA) at blood draw = (iron storage) + (0.161*EGA)

b. Babies lengths at birth [cm], n=894, R^2= 34%

	B	S. E.	Beta	T	Sig	Adj R^2
(Constant)	13,860	2,241		6,19	,000	
EGA at outcome [weeks]	,619	,039	,445	15,92	,000	,248
Mothers weight trim. 1 [kg]	,044	,010	,145	4,57	,000	,297
Baby sex [male=1]	,638	,120	,146	5,34	,000	,316
Height at admission [cm]	,053	,013	,129	4,17	,000	,328
Smoking yes/no [yes=1]	-,539	,142	-,111	-3,78	,000	,335
Parity (babies born) [N]	,091	,034	,079	2,71	,007	,341
TDP / Hb [ng/g] [1]	**,001**	**,000**	**,072**	**2,63**	**,009**	**,346**

[1] adjusted for gestational age at blood draw: (TDP / Hb) - (1.728*EGA)

c. Babies arm circumference at birth [cm], n= 892, adjusted R^2 = 23%

	B	S. E.	Beta	T	Sig.	Adj R^2
(Constant)	-2,141	,923		-2,32	,021	
EGA at date of outcome [weeks]	,283	,024	,364	12,05	,000	,173
Mothers weight trim. 1 [kg]	,030	,005	,178	5,84	,000	,211
Parity (babies born) [N]	,073	,021	,114	3,47	,001	,222
Smoking yes/no [yes=1]	-,212	,086	-,078	-2,46	,014	,226
Hematocrit ≥ 37.5% [yes=1]	**-,274**	**,131**	**-,062**	**-2,09**	**,037**	**,229**
Total DDT / fat [µg/g]	**-,016**	**,008**	**-,062**	**-2,00**	**,046**	**,232**

Highest hematocrit (≥ 37.5%) and fat adjusted DDT were significant negative determinants for arm circumference (**Table 3.9.4 c**). β-Carotene was positively whereas AGP, retinol, and DDT were negatively associated with babies head circumference (**Table 3.9.4 d**).

d. Babies head circumference at birth [cm], n= 892, adjusted R^2 = 28.5%

	B	S. E.	Beta	T	Sig.	Adj R^2
(Constant)	15,449	1,093		14,13	,000	
EGA at outcome [weeks]	,382	,028	,401	13,84	,000	,199
Parity (babies born) [N]	,137	,024	,174	5,72	,000	,236
Mothers weight trim. 1 [kg]	,035	,006	,172	5,90	,000	,264
β-carotene [µmol/L] *	,687	,257	,083	2,67	,008	,270
AGP >1mg/L	-,789	,272	-,084	-2,90	,004	,275
Retinol [µmol/L] *	-,343	,120	-,086	-2,86	,004	,280
a-Tocopherol [µmol/L] *	,018	,008	,066	2,17	,030	,283
Total DDT / fat [µg/g]	-,019	,009	-,060	-2,01	,045	**,285**

*adjusted for EGA at blood draw: β-carotene + (0.001*EGA); retinol + (0.003 *EGA); a-tocopherol - (0.449*EGA)

To account for the significant change during gestation, iron parameters, serum micronutrients and DDT residues in individual trimesters were assessed as determinants for birth outcomes. Separate 1st (n=103) and 2nd trimester (n=445) didn't show any micronutrient nor DDT as a significant predictor of pregnancy outcome variables. But the assessment of micronutrient levels in ≤ 2nd trimester (either 1st or 2nd trimester, n=546, median gestational age of 19 weeks) revealed that serum α-tocopherol was positively associated with birth weight; TDP (per volume and per hemoglobin, both unadjusted as well as EGA adjusted) and iron storage (after exclusion of TDP) were positive predictors of infants lengths; β-carotene (un-adjusted and EGA adjusted) was again a positive determinant for head circumference and AGP was negatively associated with both arm- and head circumference (**Table 3.9.5 a-e**).

Table 3.9.5 Pregnancy outcomes in relation to infection markers and blood micronutrient in 1st to 2nd trimester (≤ 2nd trimester)

a. Birth weight [gram] n=546, R^2=46.1%

	B	S. E.	Beta	T	Sig.	Adj R^2
(Constant)	-5445,39	541,47		-10,06	,000	
EGA at outcome [weeks]	158,85	9,30	,549	17,08	,000	,366
Mothers weight - trimester1 [kg]	13,20	2,32	,206	5,68	,000	,438
Height at admission [cm])	9,58	3,08	,111	3,111	,002	,445
Parity [N babies born before]	25,73	8,50	,097	3,03	,003	,453
Baby sex [male=1]	77,08	30,29	,080	2,54	,011	,458
α-Tocopherol [µmol/L] *	6,64	3,09	,068	2,15	,032	,461

adjusted for EGA at blood draw α-tocoph adj: x -(0.449*EGA) µmol/L

b. Infants lengths [cm] n=493, R^2=34%

	B	S. E.	Beta	T	Sig.	Adj R^2
(Constant)	16,97	2,115		8,02	,000	
EGA at outcome [weeks]	,694	,054	,475	12,78	,000	,263
Mothers weight trim. 1 [kg]	,079	,012	,253	6,80	,000	,320
Baby sex [male=1]	,611	,173	,130	3,53	,000	,333
TDP / hemoglobin [ng/g]	**,002**	**,001**	**,110**	**2,99**	**,003**	**,344**

c. Infants lengths [cm] n=493 (after exclusion of TDP/hb), adj.R^2=34%

	B	S. E.	Beta	T	Sig.	Adj. R^2
(Constant)	16,88	2,137		7,89	,000	
EGA at outcome [weeks]	,707	,055	,484	12,98	,000	,263
Mothers weight trim. 1 [kg]	,080	,012	,254	6,79	,000	,320
Baby sex [male=1]	,575	,173	,123	3,33	,001	,333
Iron storage [mg/kg BW]	**,053**	**,026**	**,076**	**2,05**	**,041**	**,337**

d. Babies arm circumference at birth [cm], n= 492, adj.R^2 = 30%

	B	S. E.	Beta	T	Sig.	Adj. R^2
(Constant)	-4,589	1,123		-4,09	,000	
EGA at outcome [weeks]	,352	,029	,467	12,10	,000	,250
Mothers weight trim. 1 [kg	,025	,006	,156	4,02	,000	,279
Parity [N babies born before]	,089	,026	,133	3,48	,001	,295
AGP > 1g/L [yes=1]	**-,482**	**,232**	**-,079**	**-2,07**	**,039**	**,300**

e. head circumference [cm], n=493, R^2=28%

	B	S. E.	Beta	T	Sig.	Adj. R^2
(Constant)	14,34	1,459		9,82	,000	
EGA at outcome [weeks]	,401	,037	,416	10,70	,000	,204
Parity [N babies born before]	,168	,033	,197	5,08	,000	,244
Mothers weight trim. 1 [kg]	,035	,008	,170	4,33	,000	,269
β-Carotene [µmol/L]	,862	,360	,094	2,40	,017	,279
AGP > 1g/L [yes=1]	**-,636**	**,302**	**-,081**	**-2,10**	**,036**	**,284**

Elevated AGP was a marginal significant predictor of lower birth weight (B= -148 gram, p=0.07); further iron storage (B=0.035 cm/ mg/kg BW, p=0.052) and male infant (B=0.226 cm, p=0.055) were marginally significantly and positively associated with head circumference.

In trimester 3 iron storage (un-adjusted and EGA adjusted), high hematocrit and DDT were inversely associated with birth weight (**Table 3.9.6 a**). Neither TDP nor any other micronutrient in 3rd trimester was a significant predictor of newborns lengths; high hematocrit (≥ 37.5%: -0.57 cm) and elevated AGP (>1mg/L: -1.74 cm) showed marginal significant (p<0.1) inverse associations with infants lengths. High hematocrit, DDT and iron storage in 3rd trimester were negative predictors of arm circumference (**Table 3.9.6 b**). Serum retinol and elevated AGP were negatively while β-carotene in trimester 3 was positively associated with infants head circumference (**Table 3.9.6 c**).

Table 3.8.7 Pregnancy outcomes in relation to infection markers and blood micronutrient in trimester 3

a. birth weight n=443, R^2=35%

	B	S. E.	Beta	T	Sig.	Adj. R^2
(Constant)	-2603,18	435,65		-5,98	,000	
EGA at outcome [weeks]	129,14	11,06	,458	11,68	,000	,248
Mothers weight trim. 1 [kg]	13,80	2,45	,220	5,64	,000	,301
Hematocrit ≥ 37.5% [yes=1]	-245,02	65,63	-,144	-3,73	,000	,320
Iron storage [mg/kg BW]	-13,89	4,66	-,115	-2,98	,003	,333
Smoking [yes=1]	-122,93	38,68	-,124	-3,18	,002	,344
total DDT / fat [µg/g]	-9,05	4,12	-,086	-2,19	,029	,349

b. Infant arm circumference [cm], n=401

	B	S. E.	Beta	T	Sig.	Adj. R^2
(Constant)	,280	1,419		,198	,843	
EGA at outcome [weeks]	,223	,036	,282	6,166	,000	,109
Mothers weight trim. 1 [kg]	,037	,008	,214	4,713	,000	,155
total DDT / fat [µg/g]	-,045	,013	-,153	-3,380	,001	,174
Hematocrit ≥ 37.5% [yes=1]	-,630	,210	-,135	-3,007	,003	,190
Smoking [yes=1]	-,327	,123	-,121	-2,661	,008	,202
Iron storage [mg/kg BW], adj.[1]	-,037	,015	-,113	-2,516	,012	,212

[1] iron storage adjusted = (iron storage) + (0.161*EGA at blood draw)

c. Infant head circumference [cm], n=399

	B	S. E.	Beta	T	Sig.	Adj. R^2
(Constant)	15,937	1,608		9,91	,000	
EGA at outcome [weeks]	,374	,041	,398	9,1	,000	,195
Mothers weight trim. 1 [kg]	,038	,009	,187	4,27	,000	,231
Parity [N babies born]	,132	,031	,185	4,22	,000	,254
Retinol [µmol/L] [1]	-,488	,160	-,134	-3,05	,002	,263
AGP >1mg/L	-1,851	,720	-,112	-2,57	,011	,275
β-Carotene [µmol/L] [1]	,635	,322	,086	1,97	,049	,280

(retinol) +(0.003 *EGA);   (b-carorene) + (0.001*EGA)

Except an inverse relation between negative iron storages and LBW (or positive association between iron stores and LBW), neither serum DDT nor any micronutrient had a significant impact on the prevalence of LBW and intra-uterine growth retardation (IUGR). Negative iron stores during pregnancy and iron deficiency (ferritin <12 or sTfR>8.5) in 3rd trimester reduced the risk of LBW (Exp(B)=0.46, p=0.03; Exp(B)=0.302, p=0.002). Further hematocrit levels ≥37.5% compared to <37.5%

during pregnancy (hemoglobin $\geq$125g/L, n=118/991) and in 3rd trimester (n=52/443) increased the risk of LBW (Exp(B)=2.16, p=0.008 and Exp(B)=3.35, p=0.004, respectively).

Overall, α-tocopherol, TDP and β-carotene were positive predictors of infant's weight, lengths and head circumference, respectively. Smoking and DDT residues were negative determinants for pregnancy outcome measures. High iron storage in $\leq 2^{nd}$ trimester was positively associated with newborns lengths and head circumference whereas high hematocrit, iron storage and DDT residues in 3rd trimester were negative predictors of both infants birth weight and arm circumference. Elevated AGP at any time during pregnancy was negatively associated with newborn's anthropometry.

4. Discussion and Conclusion

The overall aim of this thesis was to characterize the status and changes in iron, thiamine and micronutrients as well as exposure to DDT during pregnancy and in the post partum period. Since 2004, 2 cross sectional surveys where iron, micronutrient and DDT concentrations were measured have enrolled more than 1,000 refugee camp women and prospectively followed their pregnancies so that birth weight data has been obtained on 95% of the cohort. Furthermore sampling in the 3 month post partum period on more than 600 women for blood and breast milk has allowed comparison of the pregnancy and post-partum results. These studies have confirmed that:

1. Iron status, serum retinol, zinc, and β-carotene decreased during pregnancy. Retinol and zinc were higher in post partum than in early pregnancy whereas iron status and serum β-carotene were significantly lower. Whole blood thiamine increased with the number of weeks the supplement was provided and was still high at 12 weeks post partum. α-Tocopherol and copper increased concurrently with serum cholesterol and triglycerides during pregnancy and were significantly lower in post partum. Breast milk levels of iron, thiamine and micronutrients (retinol, β-carotene) except zinc were positively correlated to their respective blood levels in post partum.

2. Provision of thiamine improved whole blood indices reflecting good compliance to the supplement being able to compensate thiamine deficient diet in the camp. The prevalence of iron deficiency is still high despite the provision of ferrous sulphate suggesting inadequate dietary sources of iron and a low acceptance to iron supplements.

3. Religious group appears to be an important association with certain micronutrient deficiencies and this make programmatic changes difficult and different groups will need specifically targeting. Deficiency of zinc but not of vitamin A seemed to be a severe public health problem. Additional zinc supplements or zinc-enriched food rations might reduce the high prevalence of zinc deficiency in Maela camp. The introduction of micronutrient enriched flour (MEF) had a promising early effect improving both iron and zinc status in the first followed post partum women. Two years later serum zinc in pregnancy and

serum zinc and iron status in post partum were significantly higher than before the introduction of the MEF.

4. DDT residues are still highly prevalent and found in the blood of all pregnant and post partum women. The levels showed a decreasing trend during the surveys and were lower than those reported from the same area in 1998. However DDT residues were highly predicted by years of staying in the camp and remained an independent negative predictor of mean birth weight after controlling for covariates.

5. Multiple regression analyis on pregnancy outcomes revealed that blood levels of α-tocopherol were positively whereas high iron status, highest hematocrit, elevated AGP and DDT residues during pregnancy were found to be negatively associated with newborns weight. Whole blood thiamine had a significant positive impact on infant's lengths. Serum β-carotene and α-tocopherol were positively whereas serum retinol, DDT and AGP >1g/L were negatively associated with newborns head circumference

All pregnant women were provided with additional supplementary food rations (mung beans, dried fish) and supplements of thiamine, folic acid and iron while attending the weekly antenatal care consultations. At delivery all women received a single dose of vitamin A. In the post partum period additional supplementary food rations and thiamine supplements were still provided.

For the assessment of micronutrients in blood of pregnant women physiological alterations such as hemodilution (serum volume expansion) and the hyperlipidemic state during pregnancy need to be considered (Ladipo 2000, Seshadri 2001, Black 2001). Serum retinol and zinc decrease while copper and vitamin E are known to increase during gestation. To make the analysis more complex, concurrent micronutrient deficiencies and interactions between micronutrients are numerous. Vitamin A contributes to anemia by interfering with iron utilization and seems itself to be sequestered in the liver during iron deficiency; high doses of iron by supplements may interfere with the absorption of zinc and could therefore induce zinc deficiency, which alters vitamin A metabolism by depressing the formation and release of retinol-binding protein from the liver (Suharno 1992, 1993, Christian 1998, O'Brien 2000).

4.1 Retinol, α-tocopherol and carotenoids in pregnancy and post partum

Retinol and α-tocopherol in serum of pregnant and post partum women were highly correlated with serum cholesterol and triglycerides; serum β-carotene was also positively associated with cholesterol but negatively associated with triglycerides in both pregnant and post partum women. Fat soluble vitamins in breast milk including the carotenoids β-cryptoxanthin, lycopene, lutein and zeaxanthin were highly predicted by milk fat (triglycerides in breast milk).

Mean serum retinol, α-tocopherol and β-carotene were higher than respective levels for pregnant women from a previous study in Maela or reported from Nepal (Stuetz, 2006, Christian 2006, Yamini 2001) and in accordance to levels reported for pregnant and breastfeeding women from Northeast Thailand, Ethiopia, South Africa, Spain, and The Netherlands (Andert 2006, Wondmikun 2005, Papathakis 2007, Cikot 2001). The strong effect by hemodilution (serum volume expansion) especially in later pregnancy as well as the high demand of the foetus at the expense of the mother explains the significant decrease of mean retinol from 2nd to 3rd trimester despite the increase of cholesterol and triglycerides. Elevated acute phase proteins (CRP, AGP) and blood samples collected in 2nd survey (PW2, PP2 in 2006/7) were associated with lower retinol. The "DDT-induced" increase of retinol as recently described in pregnant Karen (Stuetz 2006) was not obvious in the present study. Nevertheless the fact that in 2006/7 both retinol and DDT were significantly lower than in 2004 suggests less impact by DDT residues on retinoid metabolism and as a confounding for serum retinol. The high supplemental dose of retinyl palmitate after delivery and the higher hematocrit resulted in a significantly higher serum retinol at 12 weeks post partum than in trimester 1.

Serum α-tocopherol increased progressively during pregnancy as did cholesterol and triglycerides and returned in the post partum period to 1st trimester levels. The difference of mean α-tocopherol levels between trimesters completely disappeared after adjustment for total serum fat, a phenomenon earlier described in Dutch and Spanish pregnant women (Oostenbrug 1998, Herrera 2004). α-Tocopherol might increase for the compensation of enhanced oxidative stress during hyperlipidemia (Wang 1991, deVriese 2001). Lower levels of vitamin E were associated with preeclampsia in Northern Nigeria (Ziari 1996).

The considerable range of fat adjusted serum α-tocopherol in each trimester (<2 up to 5 µmol/g fat) and in the post partum group (< 1.5 and > 3.5 µmol/g fat) indicate additional predictors for α-tocopherol beside cholesterol and triglycerides. Parity was inversely related to fat adjusted serum α-tocopherol in pregnancy, and smoking was negatively associated with α-tocopherol and fat adjusted α-tocopherol in pregnant and post partum women. The negative association between smoking and α-tocopherol could be attributed to differences in dietary intake between smokers and non-smokers or to oxidatively induced degradation of α-tocopherol as has been reported for antioxidant micronutrients (Alberg 2002, Gamble 2005). Significantly higher α-tocopherol, fat adjusted α-tocopherol, and triglycerides in 2007 (PW2, PP 2) than in 2004 (PW1, PP, PP1) is most likely the positive consequence of the increased amount of vegetable oil (additional 250 ml soybean oil weekly during antenatal care) provided since February 2005.

Serum β-carotene decreased with increasing trimester and was slightly lower in post partum than in trimester 1. The fact that in 2006/7 serum β-carotene was significantly lower in pregnant but significantly higher in post partum women than in respective groups in 2004 suggests an impact by season and therefore different availability of β-carotene containing food. Serum or plasma carotenoids have been found to be biomarkers reflecting recent vegetable and fruit intake (Campbell 1994). Maternal dietary intakes were positively correlated with plasma β-carotene in early pregnancy, at delivery and in cord blood (Scaife 2006). Season, gravidity, age and HIV infection were independent predictors of serum β-carotene among pregnant women living in Harare, Zimbabwe (Friis 2001). The highest mean post partum serum β-carotene in 2007 is most likely due to the fact that blood samples were collected in the end of the dry season (March to May) when β-carotene-rich Mango fruits are easily available. Interestingly, serum β-carotene showed in comparison to retinol and α-tocopherol an inverse correlation to serum triglycerides during pregnancy and in post partum and had a higher impact on breast milk β-carotene than did the milk fat concentration of the respective sample.

The significant positive correlations between retinol, α-tocopherol, β-carotene or lipid adjusted α-tocopherol in pregnancy and their respective serum levels in post partum suggests the impact by life style, social background and religious group; women who had a low or deficient serum level in a fat soluble vitamin during pregnancy were at high risk to have a low or deficient post partum serum level of the respective vitamin.

Muslims had significantly lower serum retinol and β-carotene (in pregnancy and post partum) than Buddhists or Christians, and Buddhists had significantly lower mean fat adjusted α-tocopherol than Muslims or Christians. The positive association between smoking and serum retinol is most likely confounded by age and religious group: mean age of the smokers was significantly higher than of non-smokers, and smokers were mainly present in the group of Buddhists. Smoking dropped out of the model assessing retinol after inclusion of religious groups (smoking was no longer a significant determinant for retinol but was still inversely correlated with α-tocopherol and β-carotene after adjustment for religion group). Body mass index, tobacco use and alcohol consumption were reported as non-dietary factors for higher serum retinol but lower concentration of antioxidant carotenoids (Roidt 1988, Pamuk 1993). Lower plasma β-carotene and significantly higher γ-tocopherol in smokers and passive smokers than in non-smokers remained significant after adjustment for triacylglycerol, race, age, BMI, and dietary intake of alcohol, fruit and vegetable (Dietrich 2003); and interestingly, higher mean plasma retinol among smokers than passive smokers was no longer significant after adjustment for dietary intakes and other covariates.

We do not have precise information of maternal diet regarding frequency of intake of fruits, vegetables and meat in the present study. However, the association between smoking and the fat soluble vitamins retinol, α-tocopherol and β-carotene is most likely to be attributed to the significantly higher age among smokers and the differences in food and smoking habits between religious groups. Furthermore owing a garden and animals were associated with higher retinol and β-carotene, and season seemed to have a strong impact on serum and milk β-carotene.

Mean concentrations of retinol and carotenoids in breast milk samples were in the range of well-nourished healthy mothers from Australia, Canada, China, Japan, the United Kingdom, Mexico, and the United States (Canfield 2003). Milk retinol was higher than reported for Karen and Lahu hill tribes (<0.8 µmol/L) from Chiang Mai province, Thailand (Panpanich 2002). Mean milk α-tocopherol was lower than reported for well-nourished Japanese women between 90-180 days post partum (Sakurai 2005, Kamao, 2007) but higher than in breast milk of Spanish mothers at day 40 of lactation (Ortega, 1999). The great variations in the results of studies on fat soluble vitamins in human milk depends on several contributing factors including differences in stage of lactation, milk fat concentrations and breast milk collection technique. Retinol, β-carotene and α-tocopherol levels are highest in colostrum and decrease in transitional milk and as the duration of lactation increases (Schweigert 2004, Sakurai 2005). Retinol and α-tocopherol have been positively associated with milk fat but not to maternal intake, and both vitamins and milk fat were significantly higher in hindmilk than in foremilk (Bishara 2008).

The variability of retinol and α-tocopherol in breast milk samples of the present study were highly predicted by milk fat concentrations (accounting for 30 and 35%, respectively). The proportions of low or deficient milk retinol (<1.05 μmol/L) decreased considerably (from 28-53% to 4.5-17%) using the milk fat adjusted cut-off (<28 μmol/kg fat). Overall, vitamin A deficiency seemed not to be a severe public health problem in Maela camp. Intake of oil is high and Vitamin A supplements after delivery are partially supervised. Liquid based as well as fat adjusted breast milk levels of lutein-zeaxanthin were much higher than those of β-cryptoxanthin and β-carotene and as high as previously reported for well nourished Japanese and Chinese mothers (Canfield 2003). Higher proportion and milk concentration of lutein-zeaxanthin than of β-carotene was also reported in Tanzanian women (Lietz 2006); the authors demonstrated a regulated uptake of the polar carotenoids lutein and zeaxanthin into breast milk indicating their requirement as protective antioxidants in infants retinal pigment epithelium. In the present study milk fat adjusted retinol, lutein-zeaxanthin and β-cryptoxanthin didn't differ between post partum groups or year of sampling. But α-tocopherol and β-carotene were still higher in 2007 than in 2004 when the levels were adjusted for milk fat; this fact confirms the positive impact by the increased provision of sunflower oil and the implication of season associated with availability of Mango fruits and/or other β-carotene rich vegetables and fruits. Concentrations of β-carotene in milk were strongly affected by respective post partum serum levels which had a higher impact on milk β-carotene than did the milk fat. The positive association between maternal diet and serum and milk β-carotene has been described in several studies (Canfield 1997, Lietz 2001, Meneses 2005, de Azeredo 2008). The intake of β-carotene-rich vegetables, oils and fruits are recommended in order to meet the vitamin A requirement for mothers and their breast fed infants whose diet excludes the consumption of meat, liver and eggs (Strobel 2007).

82

4.2 Thiamine status in pregnant and post partum women

Whole blood thiamine diphosphate (TDP) per volume and per hemoglobin increased during pregnancy and was significantly higher in post partum women. A longitudinal study in Dutch women revealed a gradual decline of total thiamine in whole blood during pregnancy and higher "pre-conceptional" concentrations at 6 weeks post partum (Cikot 2001). Mean total thiamine in whole blood increased only slightly from 1st to 3rd trimester in women from New Jersey who were daily supplemented with a vitamin-mineral pill containing 3 mg thiamine (Baker 2002), and reached about 70% of the levels measured in well-nourished, non-supplemented, non-pregnant females. In the present study, mean levels and ranges of TDP during pregnancy (109, 25-298 nM) and in post partum (126, 43-259 nM) were in the upper range of those reported for adult females of Japan (105, 50-200 nM; Ihara, 2005) and Norway (121 ± 39 nM; Tallaksen 1991) and for healthy Italian (115 ± 25 nM; Floridi 1984) and Dutch volunteers (120 ± 18; Brunnekreeft 1989).

Multivariate regression analysis revealed that highest hematocrit levels, higher mother's age and increased weeks of provided thiamine supplement were positively whereas smoking and higher parity were negatively associated with whole blood TDP during pregnancy. The significant increase of whole blood TDP with increasing trimester and total number of provided supplements until date of blood draw reflects the effectiveness and good compliance of thiamine supplementation. Significantly lower TDP in trimester 3 of women who chewed betel nut (areca) or smoked cheroots than in those who did not reflects the inhibition of thiamine absorption by betel nut consumption and possible implication by smoking. Women who smoked were significantly older (29.5 vs. 25 years) and had a higher proportion of betel nut consumers (45 vs. 15%) than non-smokers. Therefore, either the cheroots, women's age or the association between smokers and betel nut consumers are responsible for significantly lower TDP in smokers. Karen women smoke Burmese cheroots (known locally as *Kye Lah),* a kind of cigar which is approximately 15 cm in length and consists of a white dried betel nut leaf wrapper filled with coarse ground tobacco and a filter made from a blended herb (*Ahm way*) that gives a sweet taste to the smoke (McGready 1998). They usually smoke and eat betel nut particularly after their two main meals, which could explain the inhibition of thiamine absorption by both ingredients of the cheroots and betel nut chewing. Further, smoking as well as betel nut consumption was inversely associated with hemoglobin which highly predicted TDP in pregnant and post partum women. However, very low whole blood TDP within each subgroup, non-smokers or those who never chewed betel nut, suggests that failing to take the supplement had a much higher impact on thiamine status than the fact of smoking or chewing betel nut. In north-eastern Thailand betel nut chewing as well as the consumption of raw fermented fish resulted in a biochemical thiamine deficiency even in the presence of adequate thiamine intakes (Vimokesant 1975). In Maela camp, the regular consumption of nya-u htee did not affect thiamine status suggesting that the thiaminase in the fermented fish sauce was already destroyed by cooking. Overall a good compliance to high dose thiamine supplements (100 mg daily compared to recommended daily nutrient intakes (RNI) for thiamine of 1.4 and 1.5 mg for pregnant and lactating women, respectively, FAO/WHO 2001) seemed to eclipse the possible implication by betel nut, nya-u htee or smoking as 'anti-thiamine' factors.

Higher whole blood TDP in post-partum is the consequence of the ongoing thiamine supplementation and the significantly higher hemoglobin after delivery. Significantly higher thiamine in both whole blood and breast milk of Christians than of Muslim and Buddhist is most likely due to a more regular intake of provided thiamine supplements among Christians. However, significantly lower post partum TDP in 2007 than in 2004 suggest a decreased intake of thiamine in post partum women.

Thiamine, thiamine mono-phosphate and their sum as total thiamine in breast milk were highly positively correlated with whole blood TDP and depended obviously on dietary intake and thiamine status of the mother. The present study demonstrates for the first time that thiamine in human milk consists both non-phosphorylated 'free' thiamine as well as the phosphorylated form thiamine mono-phosphate (TMP), which contributed between 10 and 90% with a mean of 57% to total thiamine. A similar ratio was analysed in breast-milk samples collected in Stuttgart (n=5, own research). Monophosphate as the only thiamine phosphoric ester with an amount of about 60% of total thiamine was found in the cerebrospinal fluid of different mammals including human (Rindi 1981). Thiamine mono-phosphate (TMP) in breast milk was never reported in previous studies because thiamine was either analysed by microbiological assays or by HPLC after enzymatic hydrolysis of the thiamine esters. Mean levels of TMP and thiamine in breast-milk was highest in those mothers (PP1) who were for the first time provided with the enriched flour suggesting an additional impact despite the delivery of high dose thiamine supplements. Prentice et al (1983) reported an increase of milk thiamine (from 480 to 660 nM) in Gambian nursing mothers after providing thiamine containing supplements (1.36 mg B1/day). In the present study the mean total thiamine in milk (753 nM or 254 µg/L) was higher than reported for European (300-600 nM or 100-200 µg/L; Dostalova 1988) and vitamin supplemented (1.7 mg B1/ day), well-nourished American mothers (238 µg/L; Nail 1980). Similar amounts of thiamine were measured in mature breast-milk of Saudi women (800 nM; Al-Othman 1996). Most important in the present study is the significantly positive correlation between thiamine levels in whole blood and breast milk of the mothers. This finding demonstrates that a successful thiamine supplementation of the mothers is able to prevent breast-fed infants from thiamine deficiency and infantile beriberi, pertinent in this population given the previous catastrophic infant mortality rate at approximately 3 months of age from infantile Beri-Beri (Luxemburger et al. 2003).

In summary high mean thiamine levels in blood and milk and a simultaneously low rate of thiamine deficiency compared to available reference values indicate a high compliance to provided thiamine supplements. In 2004 micronutrient enriched flour showed an additional positive impact on thiamine levels in blood and breast milk 3-5 months after its introduction. But the significantly lower whole blood TDP in post partum two years later in 2006/7 suggests a trend towards lower dose or lower compliance to thiamine supplements amongst post partum women.

4.3 Iron status, anemia, zinc and copper during pregnancy and in post partum

The present study shows a significant decrease of serum ferritin (SF) and hematocrit levels and an inversely increase of soluble transferrin receptor (sTfR) during pregnancy. The prevalence of iron deficiency (ID defined as SF <12 µg/L or sTfR >8.5 mg/L), negative iron storage (calculated milligrams of iron reserves per kilogram body weight < 0) and of iron deficiency anemia (IDA: ID & hemoglobin < 105 in 2nd or < 110 g/L in 3rd trimester) increased significantly between 2nd and 3rd trimester; women in 3rd trimester were associated with a considerable high incidence of iron deficiency (39%), negative iron storage (23%) and iron deficiency anemia (26%) despite the provision of highly concentrated iron supplements (600 mg ferrous sulphate per day). SF rose again in post partum but sTfR and the proportion of ID (38%) in postpartum women was still as high as in trimester 3 indicating depleted iron stores after delivery.

Decreasing SF levels during pregnancy indicate the deterioration in iron stores with gestational age while the simultaneous increase of sTfR is most likely due to increased erythropoiesis and a concurrent development of tissue iron deficiency. Low SF in combination with high sTfR levels in late pregnancy was reported in iron supplemented Indonesian as well as in well-nourished low dose iron supplements consuming Swedish and American women (Carriaga 1991, Akesson 1998, 2002, Muslimatun 2001). Recent studies in Europe indicated that the incidence of iron deficiency among pregnant women was in the region of 20-40% (Bergmann, 2002, Massot, 2003). The prevalence of anemia during pregnancy in Maela is lower than reported for India or Nepal (Agarwal 2006, Dreyfuss 2000) but higher than in Bangkok, Thailand (Chotnopparatpattara 2003). Similar prevalence of anemia and iron deficiency anemia (IDA) were reported for rural Bangladesh (Hyder 2004).

The high prevalence of IDA during pregnancy in Maela despite the provision of high doses of ferrous sulphate suggests a low compliance to iron supplements or another significant source of iron loss such as intestinal helminthes, particularly hookworm. Daily iron supplementation (60 mg) in anemic pregnant women can be effective as shown in Northern Pakistan where hemoglobin and ferritin increased with duration of iron supplementation (Mumtaz 2000). Neither weekly nor daily iron-folic acid supplementation under non-supervised conditions provided enough iron to meet the needs in the third trimester of Vietnamese pregnant women who received only few or no iron-folic supplement before pregnancy (Berger 2005). In a prospective study among Peruvian women who received daily iron (60mg) and folic acid (250 µg) serum ferritin concentrations increased throughout pregnancy only in women with initial hemoglobin < 95 g/L, the risk of anemia decreased with the number of supplements consumed, and women with initial hemoglobin >95 g/L showed increases in serum ferritin by the end of pregnancy (Zavaleta 2000). Therefore benefits on maternal iron-hematologic status from iron supplementation depend on maternal iron-hematologic status in early pregnancy. Zavaleta et al. summarized the results from past placebo-controlled trials of iron supplementation as following: 1. Regardless of supplemen-tation, both hemoglobin and serum ferritin drop to the end of 2nd trimester because of hemodilution as well as other physiological changes during pregnancy. 2. Hemoglobin and serum ferritin concentrations do not rise again at the end of pregnancy without supplemental iron, even in women with adequate iron stores at the beginning of pregnancy. 3. Among women entering pregnancy with anemia (hemoglobin <110g/L), both hemoglobin and serum ferritin concentrations may rise continually throughout pregnancy, but only if supplemental iron is provided. 4. Despite iron supplementation, 10-60% of women entering prenatal care with anemia will still have anemia at the end of pregnancy. 5. Among non-anemic women at entry into prenatal care, 10-20% are likely to become anemic and 10-50% are likely to have iron deficiency by the end of pregnancy.

Low compliance to iron supplements in Maela could be due to adverse side effects of the high dose of 200 mg elemental ferrous iron (600 mg ferrous sulphate). High iron content is associated with high rates of gastrointestinal symptoms including nausea, vomiting and constipation. In one report, significantly higher non compliance (60% vs. 15%) to ferrous sulphate in daily iron (100 mg iron/day) compared to the weekly iron supplementation group (200 mg iron/week) was mainly due to gastrointestinal side-effects (Mukhopadhyay 2004). The common occurrence of nausea and vomiting in pregnancy led women to discontinue taking supplements with high levels of iron. Lower iron content of 35 mg has significantly decreased constipation rates by 30% and showed no association to the severity of nausea and vomiting as compared to higher concentrations of iron supplements with 60 mg iron (Ahn 2006). Another report demonstrated compliance to iron supplementation among pregnant women was negatively affected by side-effects and disliking the taste resulting in lower hemoglobin concentrations (Lutsey 2007).

The low intake of heme food such as meat, low intake of potential enhancers of non-heme iron absorption such as ascorbic acid as well as parasitic infections (helminths) are most likely contributing risk factors for IDA among pregnant women in Maela. To be Muslim was a strong predictor for lower iron status in pregnancy. As Muslims don't raise nor eat pigs, the commonest source of red meat in the camp, this is plausible. In addition, Muslims consumed less nyohtee than Christians and Buddhists; fermented fish paste (nyohtee) usually eaten together with rice and vegetables might be an important source of iron as well as of enhancers of iron absorption. Ascorbic acid and other organic acids available from fruits and fermented foods are described as enhancers of iron absorption due their ability to reduce ferric to ferrous iron (Fishman 2000, Hurrell 2002, Teucher 2004). A simple vinegar drink improved iron status among pregnant women with low iron status and in those who refused iron supplements because of its side effects (Heins 2000). An assessment of dietary patterns among Chinese pregnant women revealed a significantly lower intake of heme food such as meat and eggs as well as of green vegetables, fruits, retinol and ascorbic acid in the anemia than in the normal group (Ma 2002).

Helminth infections in particular hookworms were identified as risk factors for IDA among pregnant women in Thailand, Vietnam and Uganda (Piammongkol 2006, Aikawa 2006, Ndyomugyenyi 2008). An intervention programme consisting iron supplementation, deworming as well as information, education and communication (IEC) about anemia, iron-rich food, iron enhancers, etc. was able to improve haematological status of pregnant women in each trimester (Abel 2000).

Finally, high prevalence of thalassemia carriers and hemoglobinopathies as reported for Thailand should beside iron deficiency be taken into account as major causes of pregnancy-related anemia in Maela (Sanchaisuriya 2006, Sukrat 2006).

The present cross-sectional studies didn't reflect individual change and relationship of iron status between early and late pregnancy. But the follow-ups of women after delivery showed a strong relationship between iron status in pregnancy and post partum. Women who were identified with negative iron stores during pregnancy had a 5-fold higher risk for negative iron stores in post partum. There was considerable improvement of iron status in post partum women after the introduction of the micronutrient enriched flour (MEF); sTfR was significantly lower and iron in milk was significantly higher in PP1 than in PP indicating an improvement of tissue iron which also affected milk levels after a few months of provided MEF. Two years later tissue iron (sTfR) in post partum was still significantly lower than in post partum women who never received the flour.

Overall, prevalence of IDA in pregnant and post partum women in Maela camp could be reduced by a higher compliance to provided iron sulphate supplements and a sustainable acceptance to the enriched flour improving pre-pregnancy iron status. A survey of helminth infection is indicated. The consumption of the MEF is favourable in that way providing additional micronutrients such as vitamin C being able to improve non-heme iron absorption. In Tanzania a micronutrient-fortified powdered beverage containing 11 micronutrients was able to increase serum ferritin and hemoglobin in pregnant women with a high prevalence (61%) of anemia (Makola 2003). Another useful option to improve iron status in Maela would be the provision of a fortified food vehicle such as fish sauce which is well accepted and consumed daily in the population. The regular consumption of iron-fortified fish sauce significantly reduced prevalence of ID and IDA among Vietnamese women (Thuy 2003).

Zinc deficiency in pregnant and breast-feeding women in Maela camp was highly prevalent, reflecting dietary inadequacy, probably derived from a deficit of good food sources for zinc such as red meat and a predominantly plant-based staple food (rice, mung beans) with high amounts of phytates known to have an inhibitory effect on zinc absorption (Lönnerdal 2000). Comparable low levels of plasma zinc in pregnant and post partum women were reported from Peru and Nepal (Moser 1988, Caulfield 1999, Jiang 2005). The phenomena of decreasing zinc levels during pregnancy, which was also reported in well nourished populations, could be explained by a normal physiologic adjustment to pregnancy, a response to hormonal changes and by hemodilution (Hambridge 1983, Martin-Lagos 1998, Tamura 2000). Hotz et al. (2003) found a strong correlation between albumin and zinc (about 80% of zinc is bound to albumin) and a relatively constant ratio of serum zinc to albumin by month of pregnancy which explained the zinc variability and the decrease of zinc by hemodilution. High amounts of copper, iron or folate in the diet or given as supplements could alter zinc utilization. Several studies suggested that zinc absorption is antagonized by doses of iron which would result from competitive interaction between these elements (Hambridge 1983, 1987, Solomons 1986, O'Brien 2000). The prevalence of zinc deficiency was significantly higher among pregnant women consuming iron tablets (Salimi, 2004). Folic acid supplements also may contribute to the inhibition of intestinal zinc absorption, as suggested by Mukherjee et al. (1984). However, there seems only a weak (if any) association between iron status (ferritin, sTfR, ion storage) and serum zinc in Maela women. Zinc status in post partum women improved despite the iron in the MEF. As a preventive measure, zinc supplements together with the provided iron and folic acid tablets might be necessary. The IOM recommends zinc supplementation (< 35 mg/d) when ≥ 30 mg/d of supplemental iron is taken (IOM 1990). In addition dietary strategies to improve the content and bioavailability of zinc in predominantly plant-based diets are: 1. increasing intakes of foods with high content and bioavailability of zinc (fish, meat, boiled ground nuts) 2. Intake of foods known to enhance zinc absorption such as amino acids from fish, chicken, goat and organic acids such as citric acid produced during fermentation and 3. Germination and fermentation of plant-based foods to increase phytase activity in order to reduce phytic acid which is responsible for the inhibition of zinc (Gibson 1998).

Serum copper in pregnant Karen are consistent with those reported from USA, Nepal, India and Turkey (Hambridge 1983, Jiang 2005, Pathak 2002, Meram 2003); lower serum copper levels in late pregnancy were measured in Spanish, Greece and Albanian women (Martin-Lagos 1998, Schulpis 2004). The significant increase of serum copper with period of gestation is due to the higher levels of ceruloplasmin (copper containing carrier protein) in response to elevated maternal oestrogens (Martin-Lagos 1998). Elevated copper by means of ceruloplasmin could also be induced by iron deficiency (Gambling 2003). Serum copper in pregnant Karen showed an inverse correlation to serum ferritin and was positively correlated with sTfR, but was not significantly higher in women with anemia as described previously (Kalra 1989). Lower serum copper 12 weeks post partum was similar as reported in Nepalese and American lactating women (Moser 1988).

Febrile infections that produce an acute phase response may be associated with a decline in plasma zinc concentrations, hypercupremia and simultaneous elevation of the acute phase reactants CRP and AGP (Brown, 1998). Plasma zinc declines because of hepatic sequestration induced by cytokines stimulating the synthesis of hepatic metallothionein which binds zinc with a high affinity (Keen 1993). The rise of serum copper with inflammatory conditions and infectious disease is primarily due to the hepatic synthesis and release of ceruloplasmin, an acute phase reactant. In the present study, acute phase proteins CRP and AGP were associated with lower serum zinc and elevated serum copper. However, exclusion of cases with increased acute phase proteins made no difference to any of the described results; significant differences in zinc and copper between trimesters and post partum groups were consistent after exclusion of those women with elevated CRP or AGP.

Higher serum zinc in post partum is most likely due to the change in blood volume and the higher zinc absorption adapted to the higher demand in lactating women. Fung et al (1997) found an increase of 75% of fractional zinc absorption (FZA, measured from urinary enrichments of two stable zinc isotopes) in early lactation period (7-9 wk post partum). Interestingly, no increase in FZA was found in women who took iron supplements during lactation.

In the present study, serum zinc levels were significantly higher in pregnant and breast-feeding women who were provided with the enriched flour than those who were not. Iron in the flour seemed not to affect the zinc absorption (Davidson 1995) and both iron and zinc status were improved reflecting a benefit of the micronutrient enriched flour.

Mean zinc and copper in milk were equal in both groups; values were similar to those reported at 3 month post partum of women from Spain, USA, and India (Ortega 1997, Krebs 1995, Rajalakshmi 1980). Zinc and copper in milk were not associated with the levels measured in serum at 12 weeks post partum. Milk zinc levels were adequate despite low serum zinc of the mother suggesting an active transfer from serum or breast-milk. Krebs et al. showed in a prospective double-blind controlled trial that milk zinc concentrations declined significantly over the course of the study for all subjects but were not affected by zinc supplementation. In contrary to the present study, Ortega et al. found a significant positive relation between zinc levels in serum and those of mature milk.

Zinc deficiency might be associated with the delayed visual maturation syndrome and delayed development in Maela infants. Kirksey at al (1994) studied zinc nutriture of Egyptian women and found that plasma zinc during the second trimester explained 20% of the variation in birth weight Z scores; the performance on the Bayley motor test at 6 mo of age was negatively related to maternal intakes of plant zinc. Women supplemented with zinc had fetuses with indications of enhanced neurobehavioral development compared with those who were not (Merialdi 1998).

4.4 DDT residues and their association with pregnancy outcomes

DDT exposure is still evident in Maela camp despite the interruption of indoor residual house spraying since the year 2000 reflecting the longevity of this compound. Serum DDT residues of pregnant women in 2004 (PW1) were in a similar range as samples from Chiapas, Mexico collected in the end of the 1990s and to levels reported for pregnant women in the USA in the 1960s, when DDT use in the USA was at a peak (Stuetz 2006, Koepke 2004, Longnecker 1999, 2001). Significantly lower DDT levels in 2006/7 (PW2, PP2) than in 2004 (PW1, PP1, PP) reflects the decreasing trend of residues since the last official indoor DDT spraying. Similarly, higher serum and breast milk DDT levels than in present study were detected in mothers of northern Thailand in the 1990s (Prapamontol 1995, Stuetz 2001), and in women from a cotton-growing area in Punjab, India (Kalra 1994), and in household members living in DDT-treated dwellings from malaria endemic areas in South Africa and Zimbabwe (Bouwman 1990, 1991, 2006, Chikuni 1997).

DDT was initially introduced in 1944 by the US military as an insecticide to control malaria and other vector-borne diseases. After the World War II DDT was successfully applied around the world in vector control programmes but was also extensively used for agricultural purposes in the following decades (Tren 2001, Rogan 2005). In Thailand, DDT became the insecticide of choice for mosquito vector control after a successful pilot project from 1949 to 1951 in Chiang Mai Province. Since then malaria rates in the country have been dramatically decreased as a result of successful vector control based primarily on the use of DDT for residual house spraying (Chareonviriyaphap 2000). Due to its stability and its capacity to accumulate in adipose tissue, it is found in human tissues, and there is now not a single living organism on the planet that does not contain DDT (Turusov 2002). However, in humans, high amounts of DDT residues are only reported for occupationally exposed sprayers and populations living in areas where DDT was applied in cotton culture or to control vector borne diseases (Jensen 1983, Nhachi 1990, Yanez 2002, de Carvalho Dores 2003, Bouwman 2006).

DDT residues in pregnant and post partum women in Maela were mainly predicted by years of residence in Thailand, parity and year of sample collection, explaining >20%, >10% and >5% respectively of the variance in total serum DDT. Years in Thailand by means of living in Maela or other refugee camps along the western border of Thailand to Myanmar was highly positively associated, whereas parity with therefore potential for a higher number of months of breast feeding was inversely correlated with DDT residues; the significantly lower DDT levels in 2007 compared to 2004 is an indicator for the the interruption of DDT in-house spraying. Residence in a house that had ever been sprayed for malaria control was positively whereas total lactation was significantly negatively associated with serum DDT and DDE in pregnant women from Chiapas (Koepke 2004). During each period of lactation there will usually be a net loss of DDT from the mothers via breast milk (Slorach 1983). In Maela, first born infants from mothers who resided many years in Thailand had the highest burden of DDT residues. Highest DDT content in human milk of mothers nursing their first child and the significant decrease of serum and breast-milk DDT residues with increasing parity and time of lactation is well documented (Jensen 1983, Bouwman 1990, Romieu 2000, Stuetz 2001, Sarcinelli 2003). However, fat adjusted total serum DDT in pregnancy was highly positively correlated to respective levels in post partum and explained >80% of the variation in the several fold higher concentrations of fat adjusted DDT in breast milk. Therefore high DDT exposure in utero is associated subsequently with the highest burden of DDT for the breast fed infant. The assessment of the relationship between DDT exposure and infant development is still in progress and will be reported elsewhere.

One of the aims of the study was to assess the interaction between DDT and vitamin metabolism and to examine the effects of DDT on pregnancy outcomes. Interactions and positive correlations between serum retinol (vitamin A) and DDT as shown in our previous study at the same site were no longer obvious (Stuetz, 2006). A possible explanation for the contrasting findings is that p,p'-DDT, an indicator for acute exposure to DDT, was responsible for the DDT-induced increase of serum vitamin A (Stuetz 2006); since 1999 median serum p,p'-DDT (technical non-metabolized form of DDT) significantly decreased from 12.9 to 1.8 µg/L and the DDE/DDT ratio increased from 1.04 to 5.3 in 2006. The observed positive association between α-tocopherol and DDT residues in the present study was likely due to their strong correlation to serum fat.

The relatively high maternal total serum DDT, consisting of high p,p'-DDE but already low proportion of p,p'-DDT, didn't increase the risk for low birth weight (LBW), preterm delivery, small-for-gestational-age (SGA) or intra-uterine-growth-retardation (IUGR). But linear regression analysis on infant's birth weight revealed a significant inverse relation to serum-fat-adjusted DDT levels in pregnancy, after adjusting for gestational age at outcome, mother's 1st trimester weight and height, smoking status and sex of the baby. Further maternal lipid adjusted DDT residues were significantly negatively associated with length of gestation.

Findings regarding the relation of DDT and DDE to negative reproductive outcomes in human are inconsistent. One retrospective study (n=2380) using data from the US Collaborative Perinatal Project (CPP) in the early 1960s found steadily increasing odds ratios of preterm and SGA birth (BW <10th percentile at each week of gestation) with increasing (categories of) maternal serum DDE concentration (Longnecker 2001). Another retrospective study using data from the US Child Health and Development Study (CHDS, San Francisco Bay Area, 1959-1967) did not find any significant relations or trends between maternal DDT or DDE levels and preterm or SGA birth, birth weight or length of gestation despite higher maternal serum DDE concentrations (median DDE of 43 vs. 25 µg/L) than in the Longnecker's et al study (Farhang 2005). The authors supposed that the sample size with 420 male babies lacked power to detect an effect on preterm and SGA births. Recent studies assessing the relationship between DDT and adverse pregnancy outcomes are either too small in sample size or accompanied with very low DDT levels. Significant associations (OR) between maternal blood levels of HCH-isomers or p,p'-DDE and intra-uterine growth retardation (<10th percentile of birth weight for gestational age) were shown in a case control study (n=30 vs. 24 controls) from Lucknow, India by use of logistic regression models which had to be adjusted for maternal age and gestation age of the babies (Siddiqui 2003); in addition a significant negative association between maternal p,p'-DDE and weight of the newborns were noticed after gestational age had been accounted for. Increasing serum p,p'-DDE was associated with increased odds of spontaneous abortion (n=15 vs. 15 controls) in nulliparous Chinese textile workers (Korrik 2001). A study in an Australian population (n>800) using breast milk levels as index of exposure failed to achieve statistical significance between higher DDT or DDE contamination and reproductive outcomes among primiparous women (Khanjani 2006). The authors concluded that the range of total DDT contamination <7.5 mg/kg lipid in maternal milk not seem to pose a serious threat to human reproduction. Similar, the longitudinal birth cohort study in Salinas valley, California (CHAMACOS study 2000-2001, n=385) assessing effects by pesticides on health of pregnant women and children observed no adverse associations between maternal DDT or other organochlorine levels and birth weight, most likely due to lower DDE levels and smaller sample size than in the Longernecker et al. study (Fenster 2006).

DDT exposure in the present study, being several fold higher than in the Australian (median total DDT in breast milk 2.5 mg/kg, max 59 mg/kg lipid) or CHAMACOS study but slightly lower (median total serum DDT of 13 µg/L, max 233 µg/L) than in the Longnecker's study, seemed to be at the borderline required to demonstrate an impact on pregnancy outcomes. The decreasing trend of DDT residues as well as the simultaneous increase in birth weight by increase of mother's weight during the study period (2004-2007) probably diminished the power to detect DDT-related risk of adverse pregnancy outcomes (LBW, preterm delivery, SGA), whereas the relatively big sample size and the ongoing occurrence of high residues gave adequate power to detect significant inverse relations between continuous DDT levels and birth weight or gestational age. However, the impact by DDT residues on birth weight was less significant than that of mothers 1st trimester weight, parity, smoking status and infant's sex. Associations between parity, mother's weight or BMI, or smoking and infant's birth weight or risk of LBW are in agreement with the reproductive health literature and therefore strengthening the outcome of the present study (Muslimatun 2002, Neggers 2003). It seems reasonable to conclude that there is evidence for neither establishing nor rejecting a relationship between DDT exposure and pregnancy outcomes in Maela camp. A study undertake 5-10 years earlier, during a period of yearly DDT residual in-door spraying may have found a stronger association between DDT residues and birth weight. Howeverat that time malaria was highly prevalent (37% in pregnant women) and strongly associated with anemia and risk of LBW (Luxemburger 2001). Adverse pregnancy outcomes by DDT might be still obvious in endemic malaria areas in South Africa where it was sprayed for many years until 1999 and recently re-introduced as a vector control agent (Bouwman 2006). Chen and Rogan estimated an increase in infant deaths that might result from DDT spaying being of the same order of magnitude as the decrease of infant's death from effective malaria control (Chen 2003). In fact, the possible risk of 'lowering birth weight' by high DDT exposure seems negligible in relation to the high risk of adverse pregnancy outcomes by prenatal malaria infection. Therefore indoor residual spraying (IRS) of DDT seems justified in areas where its usage was shown to be highly effective to control malaria. The continuing role of DDT in malaria control is still in debate (Roberts 2000, Rogan 2005, Weissmann 2006). Numerous scientific reports and evidence against adverse health impacts argued against the final ban of DDT in malaria control programs (Attaran 2000, Bate 2007). The WHO supports the use of DDT and issued a clean bill of health for controlling malaria (www.who.int/mediacenter/news/releases/ 2006/re50/en/). The Stockholm Convention allows DDT for public health purposes. DDT can be used for IRS in countries where available data indicates that it can be effective towards achieving malaria target (WHO 2006, 2007).

4.5 Impact by micronutrients and DDT residues on pregnancy outcomes

Mean birth weight (3000 g), proportion of LBW (11%) and neonatal length (49 cm) in the present study were similar to those reported for Niger, Guinea-Bissau, Japan or Indonesia (Zagre 2007, Kaestel 2005, Takimoto 2005, Muslimatun 2002). Pregnancy outcome variables improved during the study period: In 2006, gestational age at delivery and newborns weight, length, arm- and head circumference were significantly higher and proportion of LBW and IUGR were significantly lower than in 2004. The predominant predictor accounting between 16 and 36% of the variability in newborn's anthropometry was gestational age at delivery. Mother's weight, height and parity and male gender of the newborn were important positive determinants whereas smoking was a negative predictor of fetal outcomes. The high impact of gestational age, maternal anthropometry, parity, and gender on newborn anthropometry as well as the association between smoking habits and increased risk for adverse birth outcomes (LBW, SGA, IUGR) is well reported in the reproductive health literature (Muslimatun 2002, Watson-Jones 2007, Suzuki 2008). Increased risk of LBW by smoking cheroots ('Burmese cigars') in Thai refugee camps including Maela has been reported (McGready 1998). Tobacco smoke contains many toxins which are thought to affect fetal growth through a variety of mechanism. Nicotine and carbon monoxide may impair fetal metabolism of leptin, carbon monoxide content reduces amount of oxygen available to the fetus, and nicotine affect fetal growth by constricting utero-placental arteries and thus reduce blood flow and oxygen delivery to fetus (Mantzoros 1997, Kalinka 2005, Kayemba-Kay's 2008). A program to reduce smoking amongst Karen pregnant women could lead to improved birth outcomes.

Higher mothers 1st trimester weight, higher serum α-tocopherol during pregnancy, decreasing DDT exposure, and recently introduced micronutrient enriched flour are most likely contributing factors for the improvement of birth weight and pregnancy outcomes in Maela camp during the 2 years study period (2004-2006/7).

Univariate analysis on birth weight and circulating micronutrients or DDT during pregnancy indicated positive associations to α-tocopherol but significant inverse correlations to DDT, serum ferritin, iron status and highest hematocrit levels. Iron status, DDT and hematocrit >37.5% as negative predictors and α-tocopherol as a positive determinant of birth weight was confirmed in multiple linear regression models which included gestational age at delivery, mother's weight, height, parity, smoking status, and baby's sex as significant covariates.

Iron deficiency has been proposed as one possible reason for severe maternal anemia associated with LBW or preterm delivery (Rasmussen 2001). On the contrary, high instead of low plasma ferritin levels during mid to late pregnancy (19-36 weeks' gestation) were inversely correlated with infant gestational age and birth weight and strongly associated with unfavorable outcomes (Goldenberg 1996, Lao 2000). High concentrations of serum ferritin in the 3rd trimester (week 28) resulting from a failure to decline but not after expected decrease of ferritin from early pregnancy was associated with an increased risk of preterm delivery and LBW (Scholl 1998). Women in the highest decile of maternal second-trimester serum ferritin experienced an increased risk of delivering before 34 completed weeks (Xiao 2002). The association between high hemoglobin (>120g/L) and an increased risk for LBW was described in low income, pregnant African-American adolescents (Chang 2003); low hemoglobin during the 3rd trimester played a protective role from having LBW. Very low hemoglobin in the first and second trimester increased the risk of preterm birth whereas very high hemoglobin during the first and second trimester was associated with increased risk of SGA (Scanlon 2000). Elevated hemoglobin or ferritin levels during pregnancy may be caused by insufficient blood volume expansion during pregnancy. In a retrospective study including different ethnic groups (>150,000 pregnancies) lowest measured hemoglobin during pregnancy of 85-95 g/L was associated with maximum mean birth weight, while lowest incidence for LBW and preterm labour occurred with a low hemoglobin of 95-105 g/L (Steer 1995). The incidence of LBW was significantly raised above 105 g/l and below 85 g/l compared to hemoglobin levels of 96-105 g/L. Severe anemia (<80 g/L) was significantly associated with increased risk of LBW and preterm delivery in pregnant women of Nepal (Bondevik 2001). By this criterion, a mid-trimester fall of hemoglobin concentration to about 100 g/l seems to be optimal for foetal growth. The explanation might by that the drop in maternal hemoglobin to concentrations commonly regarded as indicating anemia reflect "good" expansion of plasma volume and thus reduced blood viscosity which favours efficient blood flow within the placenta and vice versa (Steer 2000). A prospective cohort study among relatively well-nourished nulliparous women of the United Kingdom obtained similar results (Mathews 2004). Higher hemoglobin concentrations in late (but not in early) pregnancy and less changes in hemoglobin concentrations during pregnancy were strongly associated with lower birth weight. The authors suggested that a small decease in hemoglobin was due to low plasma volume expansion which caused poor placental blood flow and foetal growth. Very high hemoglobin might be due to reduced normal plasma expansion causing fetal stress because of reduced placental-fetal perfusion and should be regarded as an indicator of possible pregnancy complications rather than of adequate iron status (Yip 2000).

In the present study maternal serum α-tocopherol was positively related to birth weight, a finding which is consistent with prior reports (Lee 2004, Min 2006, Scholl 2006). The authors suggested that high vitamin E reflects a well balanced antioxidant defense system consisting of antioxidant enzymes and nutrients including vitamin E promoting fetal growth. Maternal vitamin E levels at delivery were significantly lower among women with term low birth weight infants and were significantly and positively associated with birth weight and head circumference (Von Mandach 1994, Masters 2007).

A non-antioxidant property of vitamin E is the up-regulation and release of prostacyclin which induce vasodilatation and regulation of blood flow between placenta and fetus (Klockenbusch 2000). Thus high serum α-tocopherol during pregnancy should promote optimal placental blood flow and fetal growth. The increasing consumption of α-tocopherol by smoking and therefore reduction in prostacyclin may explain the birth weight reduction in infants exposed in utero to cigarette smoke (Steuerer 1999). Dietary vitamin E is primarily composed of α- and γ-tocopherol, and the richest sources are edible vegetable oil (Traber 2007). Serum α-tocopherol is significantly influenced by vitamin E intake, total fat intake and BMI (Sinha 1993, Gascon-Vila 1997). In Maela, higher α-tocopherol in 2006/7 than in 2004 is most likely the positive consequence of the additional provided ration of soybean oil during antenatal care. The higher intake of oil and thus higher calorie intake might be responsible for the improvement of mother's and subsequently newborns weight. However, serum α-tocopherol during pregnancy was a positive predictor of birth weight before (PW1 in 2004) and after (PW2 in 2006/7) additional provision of soybean oil. In Caucasien women living in Bosten, USA, vitamin E intake during pregnancy, ascertained through food frequency questionnaires, had a significant positive association with birth weight after controlling for total energy intake and several non-dietary variables including gestational age at delivery, mother's anthropometry, smoking during pregnancy and gender of the baby (Lagiou 2005).

In the present study, no relation could be shown between serum zinc in pregnancy and birth weight. The explanation might be that nearly all pregnant women had zinc deficient serum levels. Neggers et al. (1990) reported a significant relation between maternal gestational-age-adjusted serum zinc and birth weight after controlling for various independent determinants (gestational age, race, pre-pregnancy weight, smoking, and sex of the infant), and a eight times higher prevalence of low birth weight among women with serum concentrations in the lowest quartile. Zinc supplementation in pregnant African American women who had low plasma zinc at admission revealed that their infants had significantly greater birth weight and head circumference than those receiving a placebo (Goldenberg 1995). But it has to be noted that most trials failed to demonstrate any impact of supplementation of zinc alone or in combination with other micronutrient on pregnancy outcomes and infants development. Whole blood thiamine-diphosphate in pregnancy was significantly associated with newborn lengths. There is no other study which assessed blood levels of thiamine during pregnancy in relation to birth outcomes. However, Ortega et al. (2004) found a positive correlation (r 0.46, $p<0.05$) between the ratio of dietary thiamine per carbohydrate intake in pregnancy and the length of the newborn infants. Recent randomized controlled trials in rural Burkina Faso showed a significant positive impact on newborn length due to prenatal provision of multiple micronutrients. Women who were provided with the UNICEF/WHO/UNO international multiple micronutrient preparation (MMN), which included thiamine, delivered babies with higher birth lenghts (+3.6 mm, $p=0.012$) than those who received iron and folic acid alone (Roberfroid 2008); a second trial showed that the provison of a fortified spread consisting of peanut butter, soyflour, sugar, vegetable oil and multiple micronutrients (with an equal composition as the MMN) to pregnant women improved mean birth length (+4.6 mm, $p=0.001$) compared to supplementation with the multiple micronutrients alone (Huybregts 2009). The thiamine content in the MMN preparation as well as in the peanut butter might have been responsible for the improvement in newborns lenghts.

In conclusion this study showed that α-tocopherol, β-carotene and TDP were positively whereas iron status, highest hematocrit, elevated AGP and DDT residues were negatively associated with newborns weight and size parameters. Iron, micronutrient and DDT levels in pregnancy may have direct effects or may be markers for other non-obvious predictors of these pregnancy outcomes. The inverse relation between high iron status, highest hematocrit levels or high serum retinol (in particular in late pregnancy) and birth weight or arm- and head circumference are most likely due to insufficient hemodilution. The positive impact by thiamine on infant's length is obviously caused by antenatal thiamine supplementation. The positive association between α-tocopherol and birth weight might be the consequence of the higher amount of provided soybean oil. The relation between β-carotene and head circumference could be related to season of survey and higher fruit or vegetable intake (Mangos in April, pumpkins and gourd in October to November). Further the antioxidant vitamins α-tocopherol and β-carotene are decreased during infection, and increased AGP as a marker of infections was inversely associated with newborns weight and size. Finally the micronutrient enriched flour consisting basic vitamins and minerals might have been involved in the improvement of pregnancy outcomes during the study period. Supplementation of multiple micronutrients in poor communities in Nepal, to under-nourished pregnant women in Delhi, India and among pregnant women in Dar es Salaam, Tanzania increased birth weight and in rural Burkina Faso increased birth lenght when compared with standard prenatal supplemental iron and folic acid (Osrin 2005, Gupta 2007, Fawzi 2007, Roberfroid 2008).

As more than one third of women of reproductive age in Maela camp are less than 150 cm the positive impact by thiamine status on newborn length is an important finding which demonstrates the supplementation of thiamine as an effective measure to improve foetal growth. One of the remaining micronutrient problems is zinc deficiency. Prenatal supplemenation should perhaps continue with the addition of zinc. Further significant efforts to determine cause and solution to iron deficiency are needed. The consumption of micronutrient enriched flour should be encouraged for a sustainable improvement of zinc and iron status in pregnant and lactating women.

Literature

Agarwal KN, Agarwal DK, Sharma A, Sharma K, Prasad K, Kalita MC, Khetarpaul N, Kapoor AC, Vijayalekshimi L, Govilla AK, Panda SM, Kumari P (2006). Prevalence of anaemia in pregnant and lactating women in India. Indian J Med Res 124: 173-184.

Ahn E, Pairaudeau N, Pairaudeau N Jr, Cerat Y, Couturier B, Fortier A, Paradis E, Koren G (2006). A randomized cross over trial of tolerability and compliance of a micronutrient supplement with low iron separated from calcium vs high iron combined with calcium in pregnant women. BMC Pregnancy and Childbirth 6: 10.

Aikawa R, Khan NC, Sasaki S, Binns CW (2006). Risk factors for iron-deficiency anaemia among pregnant women living in rural Vietnam. Public Health Nutrition 9(4): 443-448.

Akesson A, Bjellerup P, Berglund M, Bremme K, Vahter M (1998). Serum transferrin receptor: a specific marker of iron deficiency in pregnancy. Am J Clin Nutr 68: 1241-6.

Akesson A, Bjellerup P, Berglund M, Bremme K, Vahter M (2002). Soluble transferring receptor: longitudinal assessment from pregnancy to postlactation. Obstet Gynecol 99: 260-6

Alberg A (2002). The influence of cigarette smoking on circulating concentrations of antioxidant micronutrients. Toxicology 180: 121-37.

Allen LH (2005). Multiple micronutrients in pregnancy and lactation: an overview. Am J Clin Nutr 81(suppl.): 1206S-12S.

Al-Othman AA., El-Fawaz H, Hewedy FM, Al-Khalifa AS (1996). Mineral and vitamin content of mature breast milk of Saudi lactating mothers. Ecol Food Nutr 34: 327-336.

Andert CU, Sanchaisuriya P, Sanchaisuriya K, Schelp FP, Schweigert FJ (2006). Nutritional status of pregnant women in Northeast Thailand. Asia Pac J Clin Nutr 15(3): 329-334.

Attaran A, Maharaj R (2000). Doctoring malaria badly: the global campaign to ban DDT. BMJ 321: 1403-4.

Baker H, DeAnglis B, Holland B, Gittens-Williams L, Barrett T (2002). Vitamin profile of 563 gravidas during trimester of pregnancy. J Am College Nutr 21(1): 33-37.

Banjong O, Menefee A, Sranacharoenpong K, Chittchang U, Eg-kantrong P, Boonpraderm A, Tamachotipong S (2003). Dietary assessment of refugees living in camps: a case study of Mae La Camp, Thailand. Food and Nutrition Bulletin 24(4): 360-67.

Bate R (2007). The rise, fall, rise, and imminent fall of DDT. AEI outlook series, print 22368, No.14, November 2007.

Berger J, Thanh HTK, Cavalli-Sforza T, Smitasiri S, Khan NC, Milani S, Hoa PT, Quang ND, Viteri F (2005). Community mobilization and social marketing to promote weekly iron-folic acid supplementation in women of reproductive age in Vietnam: impact on anemia and iron status. Nutr Rev 63(12): S95-S108.

Bergmann RL, Gravens-Müller, Hertwig K, Hinkel J, Andres B, Bergmann KE, Dudenhausen JW (2002). Iron deficiency is prevalent in a sample of pregnant women at delivery in Germany. Eur J Obstet Gynecol & Reprod Biology 102: 155-160.

Bishara R, Dunn MS, Merko SE, Darlin P (2008). Nutrient composition of hindmilk produced by mothers of very low birth weight infants born at less than 28 weeks' gestation. J Hum Lact 24(2): 159-67.

Bondevik GT, Lie RT, Ulstein M, Gunnar Kvale (2001). Maternal haematological status and risk of low birth weight and preterm delivery in Nepal. Acta Obstet Gynecol Scand 80: 402-408.

Bouwman H, Reinecke AJ, Cooppan RM, Becker PJ (1990). Factors affecting levels of DDT and metabolites in human breast milk from KwaZulu. J Toxicol Environ Health 31: 93-115.

Bouwman H, Cooppan RM, Becker PJ, Ngxongo S (1991). Malaria control and levels of DDT in serum of two populations in KwaZulu. J Toxicol Environ Health 22: 141-155.

Bouwman H, Sereda B, Meinhardt HM (2006). Simultaneous presence of DDT and pyrethroid residues in human breast milk from a malaria endemic area in South Africa. Environ Pollut 144: 902-917.

Black RE (2001). Micronutrients in pregnancy. Br J Nutr 85 (suppl 2): S193-S197.

Brown KH (1998). Effect of infections on plasma zinc concentrations and implications for zinc status assessment in low-income countries. Am J Clin Nutr 68(suppl): 425S-9S.

Brunnekreeft JWI, Eidhof H, Gerrits J (1989). Optimized determination of thiochrome derivatives of thiamine and thiamine phosphates in whole blood by reversed-phase liquid chromatography with precolumn derivarization. J Chromatography 491: 89-96.

Campbell DR, Gross MD, Martini MC, Grandits GA, Slavin JL, Potter JD (1994). Plasma carotenoids as biomarkers for vegetable and fruit intake. Cancer Epidemiology, Biomarkers & Prevention 3: 493-500.

Canfield LM, Giuliano AR, Neilson EM; Yap HH, Graver EJ, Cui HA, Blashill BM (1997). β-Carotene in breast milk and serum is increased after a single β-carotene dose. Am J Clin Nutr 66: 52-61.

Canfield LM, Clandinin MT, Davies DP, Fernandez MC, Jackson J, Hawkes J, Goldman WJ, Pramuk K, Reyes H, Sablan B, Sonobe T, Bo Xu (2003). Multinational study of major breast milk carotenoids of healthy mothers. Eur J Nutr 42: 133-141.

Carriaga MT, Skikne BS, Finley B, Cutler B, Cook JD. Serum transferrin receptor for the detection of iron deficiency in pregnancy. Am J Clin Nutr 1991; 54: 1077-81.

Caulfield LE, Zavaleta, and Figueroa A (1999). Adding zinc to prenatal iron and folate supplements improves maternal and neonatal zinc status in a Peruvian population. Am J Clin Nutr 69: 1257-63.

CCSDPT, Committee for Coordination of Services to Displaced Persons in Thailand (2006). 2006 Annual Health Information Short Report - Thailand/Burma Border Refugee Camps.www.tbbc.org

Centers for Disease Control and Prevention (1989). Criteria for anemia in children and childbearing aged women. MMWR 38: 400-404.

Chang SC, O'Brien KO, Nathanson MS, Mancini J, Witter FR (2003). Hemoglobin concentrations influence birth outcomes in pregnant African-American adolescents. J Nutr 133: 2348-2355.

Chareonviriyaphap T, Bangs MJ, Ratanatham S (2000). Status of malaria in Thailand. Southeast Asian J Trop Med Public Health 31(2): 225-237.

Chen A, Rogan (2003). Nonmalarial infant deaths and DDT use for malaria control. Emerging Infectious Diseases 9(8): 960-964.

Chikuni O, Nhachi CFB, Nyazema NZ, Polder A, Nafstad I, Skaare JU (1997). Assessment of environmental pollution by PCBs, DDT, and its metabolites using human milk of mothers in Zimbabwe. Sci Total Environ 199:183-190.

Chotnopparatpattara P, Limpongsanurak S, Charnngam C (2003). The prevavlence and risk factors of anemia in pregnant women. J Med Assoc Thai 86 (11): 1001-6.

Cikot R, Steegers-Theunissen R, Thomas C, deBoo TM, Merkus H, Steegers E (2001). Longitudinal vitamin and homocysteine levels in normal pregnancy. Br J Nutr 85: 49-58.

Cook JD, Baynes RD, Skikne BS (1992). Iron deficiency and the measurement of iron status. Nutr Res Rev 5: 189-202.

Cook JD, Flowers CH, Skikne BS (2003). The quantitative assessment of body iron. Blood 101(9): 3359-64.

Cook JD (2005). Diagnosis and management of iron-deficiency anaemia. Best Practice and Research Clinical Haematology Vol.18. No.2: 319-332.

Christian P, West KP Jr (1998). Interactions between zinc and vitamin A: an update. Am J Clin Nutr 68 (suppl): 435S-41S.

Christian P, Jiang T, Khatry SK, LeClerq SC, Shrestha SR, West KP Jr (2006). Antenatal supplementation with micronutrients and biochemical indicators of status and subclinical infection in rural Nepal. Am J Clin Nutr 83: 788-94.

de Azeredo VB, Trugo NMF (2008). Retinol, carotenoids, and tocopherol in the milk of lactating adolescents and relationships with plasma concentrations. Nutrition 24: 133-139.

de Carvalho Dores EFG, Carbo L, de Abreu ABG (2003). Serum DDT in malaria vector control sprayers in Mato Grosso State, Brasil. Cad Saude Publica 19 (2): 1-10.

de Vriese SR, Dhont M, Christophe AB (2001). Oxidative stability of low density lipoproteins and vitamin E levels increase in maternal blood during normal pregnancy. Lipids 36(4): 361-366.

Davidson L, Almgren A, Sandström B, Hurrell RF. Zinc absorption in adult humans: the effect of iron fortification. Br J Nutr 1996; 74: 417-425.

Davis RE, Icke GC. Clinical chemistry of thiamin. Adv Clin Chem 1983; 23:93-140.

Dietrich M, Block G, Norkus EP, Hudes M, Traber M, Cross CE, Packer L (2003). Smoking and exposure to environmental tobacco smoke decrease some plasma antioxidants and increase γ-tocopherol in vivo after adjustment for dietary intakes. Am J Clin Nutr 77: 160-6.

Dubowitz LMS, Dubowitz V (1977). Gestational assessment of the newborn: a clinical manual. Reading, CA: Addison-Wesley Publishing, 1977.

Dostalova L, Salmenpera L, Vaclavinkova V, Heinz-Erian P, Schuep W (1988). Vitamin concentration in term milk of European mothers. In *Vitamins and Minerals in Pregnancy and Lactation*. Nestle Nutrition Workshop Series, Vol 16: 275-298. New York: Nestec Ldt, Vevey/Raven Press.

Dreyfuss ML, Stoltzfus RJ, Shrestha JB, Pradhan EK, LeClerq SC, Khatry SK, Shrestha SR, Katz J, Albonico M, West KP Jr (2000). Hookworms, malaria and vitamin A deficiency contribute to anemia and iron deficiency among pregnant women in the plains of Nepal. J Nutr 130: 2527-2536.

Erhardt JG, Estes JE, Pfeiffer CM, Biesalski HK, Craft NE (2004). Combined measurement of ferritin, soluble transferrin receptor, retinol binding protein, and C-reactive protein by an inexpensive, sensitive, and simple sandwich enzyme-linked immunosorbent assay technique. J Nutr 134: 3127-32.

FAO/WHO (2001). Human vitamin and mineral requirements. Report of a joint FAO/WHO expert consultation in Bangkok, Thailand. Food and Nutrition Division, FAO Rome, 2001.

Farhang L, Weintraub JM, Petreas M, Eskenazi B, Bhatia R (2005). Association of DDT and DDE with birth weight and length of gestation in the child health and development studies. Am J Epidemiol 162 (8): 1-9.

Fawzi WW, Msamanga GI, Urassa W, Hertzmark E, Petraro P, Willett WC, Spiegelman S (2007). Vitamins and perinatal outcomes among HIV-negative women in Tanzania. N Engl J Med 356: 1423-31.

Fenster L, Eskenazi B, Anderson M, Bradman A, Harley K, Hernandez H, Hubbard A, Barr DB (2006). Association of in utero organochlorine pesticide exposure and fetal growth and length of gestation in an agriculture population. Environ Health Perspect 114: 597-602.

Fishman SM, Christian P, Weszt KP Jr (2000). The role of vitamins in the prevention and control of anemia. Public Health Nutrition 3(2): 125-150.

Floridi A, Pupita M, Palmerini CA, Fini C, Fidanza AA (1984). Thiamine pyrophosphate determination in whole blood and erythrocytes by high performance liquid chromatography. Internat J Vit Nutr Res 54: 165-171.

Friis H, Gomo E, Kaestel P, Ndhlovu P, Nyazema N, Krarup H, Fleischer Michaelsen K (2001). HIV and other predictors of serum β-carotene and retinol in pregnancy: a cross-sectional study in Zimbabwe. Am J Clin Nutr 73: 1058-65.

Fung EB, Ritchie LD, Woodhouse LR, Roehl R, King JC (1997). Zinc absorption in women during pregnancy and lactation. Am J Clin Nutr 66: 80-8.

Gamble MV, Ahsan H, Xinhua L, Factor-Litvak P, Ilievski V, Slavkovich V, Parvez F, Graziano JH (2005). Folate and cobalamin deficiencies and hyper-homocysteinemia in Bangladesh. Am J Clin Nutr 81: 1372-7.

Gambling L, Danzeisen R, Fosset C, Andersen HS, Dunford S, Srai SKS, McArdle HJ (2003). Iron and copper interactions in development and the effect on pregnancy outcome. J Nutr 133 (suppl): 1554S-1556S.

Gascon-Vila P, Garcia-Closas R, Serra-Majem L, Pastor MC, Ribas L, Ramon JM, Marine-Font A, Salleras L (1997). Determinants of the nutritional status of vitamin E in a non-smoking Mediterranean poplation. Analysis of the effect of vitamin E intake, alcohol consumption and body mass index on the serum alpha-tocopherol concentration. Eur J Clin Nutr 51: 723-728.

Gerrits J, Eidhof H, Brunnekreeft JWI, Hessels J (1997). Determination of thiamin and thiamin phosphates in whole blood by reversed-phase liquid chromatography with precolomn derivatization. Methods Enzymol 279: 74-82.

Gibson RS, Yeudall F, Drost N, Mtitimuni B, Cullinan T. Dietary interventions to prevent zinc deficiency. Am J Clin Nutr 1998; 68(suppl): 484S-7S.

Goldenberg RL, Tamura T, Neggers YH, Cooper RL, Johnston KE, DuBard MB, Hauth MD (1995). The effect of zinc supplementation on pregnancy outcome. JAMA 274: 463-468.

Goldenberg RL, Tamura T, DuBard DJP et al (1996). Plasma ferritin and pregnancy outcomes. Am J Obstet Gynecol 175:1356-1359.

Gupta PC, Ray CS (2004). Epidemiology of betel quid usage. Ann Acad Med Singapore 33(Suppl): 31S-36S.

Gupta P, Ray M, Dua T, Radhakrishnan G, Kumar R, Sachdev HPS (2007). Multimicronutrient supplementation for undernourished pregnant women and the birth size of their offspring. Arch Pediatr Adolesc Med 161: 58-64.

Hambridge, KM, Krebs NF, Jacobs MA, Favier A, Guyette L, Ikle DN (1983). Zinc nutritional status during pregnancy: a longitudinal study. Am J Clin Nutr 37: 429-442.

Hambridge KM, Krebs NF, Sibley L,English J (1987). Acute effects of iron therapy on zinc status during pregnancy. Obstet Gynecol 70: 593-6.

Heins U, Koebnick C, Leitzmann C (2000). Vinegar drink to improve iron status during pregnancy. In: Trace Elements in Man and Animals 10, Part II Subpart 4: 379-380. Springer 2000.

Herrera E, Ortega H, Alvino G, Giovannini N, Amusquivar E, Cetin I (2004). Relationship between plasma fatty acid profile and antioxidants vitamins during normal pregnancy. Eur J Clin Nutr 58: 1231-1238.

Hotz C, Peerson JM, Brown KH (2003). Suggested lower cut-offs of serum zinc concentrations for assessing zinc status: reanalysis of the second National Health and Nutrition Examination Survey data (1976-1980). Am J Clin Nutr 78:756-64.

Hurrell RF (2002). How to ensure adequate iron absorption from iron-fortified food. Nutr Rev 60: S7-15.

Huybregts L, Roberfroid D, Lanou H, Menten J, Meda N, Van Camp J, Kolsteren P (2009). Prenatal food supplementation fortified with multiple micronutrients increases birth length: a randomized controlled trial in rural Burkina Faso. Am J Clin Nutr, October 2009, epub ahead of print.

Hyder SMZ, Persson LA, Chowdhury M, Lönnerdal B, Ekström EC (2004). Anaemia and iron deficiency during pregnancy in rural Bangladesh. Public Health Nutrition 7(8): 1065-70.

Ihara H, Hirano A, Wang L, Okada M, Hashizume N (2005). Reference values for whole blood thiamine and thiamine phosphate esters in Japanese adults. Journal of Analytical Bio-Science 28(3):241-246.

IOM, Institute of Medicine. Nutrition during pregnancy. Washington DC: National Academy Press, 1990.

Jensen AA (1983). Chemical contaminants in human milk. Residue Rev 89: 1-128.

Jiang T, Christian P, Khatry SK, Wu L, West Jr KP (2005). Micronutrient deficiencies in early pregnancy are common, concurrent, and vary by season among rural Nepali pregnant women. J Nutr 135: 1106-1112.

Kaestel P, Michaelsen KF; Aaby P, Friis H (2005). Effects of prenatal multimicronutrient supplementation on birth weight and perinatal mortality: a randomised, controlled trial in Guinea-Bissau. Eur J Clin Nutr 59(9).

Kalinka J, Hanke W, Sobala W (2005). Impact of prenatal tobacco smoke exposure, as measured by midgestation serum cotinine levels, on fetal biometry and umbilical flow velocity waveforms. Am J Perinatology 22(1): 41-47.

Kalra R, Kalra VB, Sareen PM, Khandelwal R (1989). Serum copper and ceruloplasmin in pregnancy with anemia. Indian J Pathol Microbiol 32(1): 28-32.

Kalra RL, Singh B, Battu RS (1994). Organochlorine pesticide residues in human milk in Punjab, India. Environ Pollut 85: 147-151.

Kamao M, Tsugawa N, Suhara Y, Wada A, Mori T, Murata K, Nishino R, Ukita T, Uenishi K, Tanaka K, Okano T (2007). Quantification of fat-soluble vitamins in human breast milk by liquid chromatography-tandem mass spectrometry. J Chromatography B 859: 192-200.

Kayemba-Kay's S, Geary MPP, Pringle J, Rodeck CH, Kingdom JCP, Hindmarsh PC (2008). Gender, smoking during pregnancy and gestational age influence cord leptin concentrations in newborn infants. Eur J Endocrinology 159: 217-224.

Keen CL, Taubeneck MW, Daston GP, Rogers JM, Gershwin ME (1993). Primary and secondary zinc deficiency as factors underlying abnormal CNS development. Ann N Y Sci 678: 3-47.

Keizer SE, Gibson RS, O'Conner DL (1995). Postpartum folic acid supplementation of adolescents: impact on maternal folate and zinc status in milk composition. Am J Clin Nutr 62: 377-84.

Kirksey A, Wachs TD, Feisek Y, Srinath U, Rahmanifar A, McCabe GP, Osman MG, Harrison GG, Jerom NW. Relation of maternal zinc nutriture to pregnancy outcome and infant development in an Egyptian village. Am J Clin Nutr 1994; 66: 782-92.

Klockenbusch W, Goecke TW, Krüssel JS, Tutscheck BA, Crombach G, Schrör K (2000). Prostacycline deficiency and reduced fetoplacental blood flow in pregnancy-induced hypertension and preeclampsia. Gynecol Obstet Invest 50: 103-7.

Koepke R, Warner M, Petreas M, Cabria A, Danis A, Hernandez-Avila M, Eskenazi B (2004). Serum DDT and DDE levels in pregnant women of Chiapas, Mexico. Arch Environ Health 59 (11): 559-65.

Korrick SA, Chen C, Damokosh AI, Ni J, Liu X, Cho SI, Altshul L, Ryan L, Xu X (2001). Association of DDT with spontaneous abortion: a case-control study. Ann Epidemiol 11(7): 491-6.

Krebs NF, Reidinger CJ, Hartley S, Robertson AD, Hambridge KM (1995). Zinc supplementation during lactation: effects on maternal status and milk zinc concentrations. Am J Clin Nutr 61: 1030-6.

Ladipo OA (2000). Nutrition in pregnancy: mineral and vitamin supplements. Am J Clin Nutr 72 (suppl). 280S-90S.

Lagiou P, Mucci L, Tamimi R, Kuper H, Lagiou A, Hsieh CC, Trichopoulos D (2005). Micronutrient intake during pregnancy in relation to birth size. Eur J Nutr 44: 52-59.

Lao TT, Tam KF, Chan LY (2000). Third trimester iron status and pregnancy outcome in non-anaemic women; pregnancy unfavourably affected by maternal iron excess. Human Reproduction 15(8): 1843-1848.

Lee BE, Hong YC, Kim YJ, Chang NS, Park EA, Park EA, Hann HJ (2004). Influence of maternal serum levels of vitamin C and E during the second trimester on birth weight and length. Eur J Clin Nutr 58: 1365-1371.

Lietz G, Henry CJK, Mulokozi G, Mugyabuso JKL, Ballart A, Ndossi GD, Lorri W, Tomkins A (2001). Comparison of the effects of supplemental red palm oil and sunflower oil on maternal vitamin A status. Am J Clin Nutr 74: 501-9.

Lietz G, Mulokozi G, Henry JCK, Tomkins AM (2006). Xantophyll and hydrocarbon carotenoid pattern in plasma and breast milk of women supplemented with red palm oil during pregnancy and lactation. J Nutr 136: 1821-1827.

Lönnerdal B (2000). Dietary factors influencing zinc absorption. J Nutr 130: 1378S-1383S.

Longnecker MP, Klebanoff MA, Gladen BC, Berendes HW (1999). Serial levels of serum organochlorines during pregnancy and postpartum. Arch Environ Health 54(2): 110-14.

Longnecker MP, Klebanoff MA, Zhou H, Brock JW (2001). Association between maternal serum concentration of the DDT metabolite DDE and preterm and small-for-gestational-age babies at birth. The Lancet 358: 110-114.

Lucas A, Hudson GJ, Simpson P, Cole TJ, Baker BA (1987). An automated enzymatic micromethod for the measurement of fat in human milk. Journal of Dairy Research 54: 487-492.

Lutsey P, Dawe D, Villate E, Valencia S, Lopez O (2007). Iron supplementation compliance among pregnant women in Bicol, Philippines. Public Health Nutrition 11(1): 76-82.

Luxemburger C, McGready R, Kham A, Morison L, Cho T, Chongsuphajaisiddhi T, White NJ, Nosten F (2001). Effects of malaria during pregnancy on infant mortality in an area of low malaria transmission. Am J Epidemiology 154(5): 459-465.

Luxemburger C, White NJ, ter Kuile F, Singh HM, Allier-Frachon I, Ohn M, Chongsuphajaisiddhi T, Nosten F (2003). Beri-beri: the major cause of infant mortality in Karen refugees. Trans R Soc Trop Med Hyg 97(2):251-5.

Ma A, Chen X, Zheng M, Wang Y, Xu R and Li J (2002). Iron status and dietray intake of Chinese pregnant women with anaemia in the third trimester. Asia Pacific J Clin Nutr 11(3): 171-175.

Mantzoros CS, Varvarigou A, Kaklamani VG, Beratis NG, Flier JS (1997). Effect of birth weight and maternal smoking on cord blood leptin concentrations of full-term and preterm newborns. J Clin Endocrinol Metab 82: 2856-61

McGready R, Simpson JA, White NJ, Nosten F, Lindsay SW (1998). Smoking cheroots reduces birth weight. The Lancet 352: 1521-22.

McGready R, Simpson JA, Cho T, Dubowitz L, Changbumrung S, Bohm V, Munger RG, Sauberlich HE, White NJ, Nosten F (2001). Postpartum thiamine deficiency in a Karen displaced population. American Journal of Clinical Nutrition 74(6):808-813.

McGready R, Simpson JA, Arunjerdja R, Golfetto I, Ghebremeskel K, Taylor A, Siemieniuk A, Mercuri E, Harper G, Dubowitz L, Crawford M, Nosten F (2003). Delayed visual maturation in Karen refugee infants. Ann Trop Paediatr 23(3): 193-204.

Makola D, Ash DM; Tatala SR, Latham MC, Ndossi G, Mehansho H (2003). A micronutrient-fortified beverage prevents iron deficiency, reduces anemia and improves the haemoglobin concentration of pregnant Tanzanian women. J Nutr 133: 1339-1346.

Martin-Lagos F, Navarro-Alarcon M, Terres-Martos C, Lopez-Garcia de la Serrana H, Perez-Valero V, Lopez-Martinez MC (1998). Zinc and copper concentrations in serum from Spanish women during pregnancy. Biol Trace Elem Res 61(1): 61-70.

Massot C, Vanderpas J (2003). A survey of iron deficiency anaemia during pregnancy in Belgium. Acta Clinica Belgica 58 (3): 169-177.

Masters ET, Jedrychowski W, Schleicher RL, Tsai W-Y, Tu Y-H, Camann D, Tang D, Perera FP (2007). Relation between prenatal lipid-soluble micronutrient status, environmental pollutant exposure, and birth outcomes. Am J Clin Nutr 86: 1139-45.

Mathews F, Youngman L, Neil A (2004). Maternal circulating nutrient concentrations in pregnancy: implications for birth and placental weights of term infants. Am J Clin Nutr 79: 103-10.

Meneses F, Trugo NMF (2005). Retinol, β-carotene, and lutein + zeaxanthin in the milk of Brazilian nursing mothers: associations with plasma concentrations and influences of maternal characteristics. Nutrition Research 25: 443-451.

Meram I, Bozkurt AI, Ahi S, Ozgur S (2003). Plasma copper and zinc levels in pregnant women in Gaziantep, Turkey. Saudi Med J 24 (10): 1121-5.

Merialdi M, Caulfield LE, Zavaleta N, Figueroa A, DiPietro JA (1998). Adding zinc to prenatal iron and folate tablets improves neurobehavioral development. Am J Obstet Gynecol 180: 483-490.

Moser PB, Reynolds RD, Acharya S, Howard MP, Andon MB, Lewis SA (1988). Copper, iron, zinc, and selenium dietary intake and status of Nepalese lactating women and their breast-fed infants. Am J Clin Nutr 47: 729-34.

Min J, Park H, Park B, Kim YJ, Park J, Lee H, Ha E, Park EA, Hong YC (2006). Paraoxonase gene polymorphism and vitamin levels during pregnancy: relationship with maternal oxidative stress and neonatal birth weights. Reproductive Toxicology 22(3): 418-24.

Muherjee MK, Sandstead HH, Ratnaparkhi MV, Johnson LK, Milne DB, Stelling HP (1984). Maternal zinc, iron, folic acid, and protein nurtiture and outcome of human pregnancy, Am J Clin Nutr 40: 496-507.

Mukhopadhyay A, Bhatla N, Kriplani A, Pandey RM, Saxena R (2004). Daily versus intermittent iron supplementation in pregnant women: Hematological and pregnancy outcome. J Obstet Gynaecol Res 30(6): 409-417.

Mumtaz Z, Shahab S, Butt N, Rab MA, DeMuynck A (2000). Daily iron supplementation is more effective than twice weekly iron supplementation in pregnant women in Pakistan in a randomized double-blind clinical trial. J Nutr 130: 2697-2702.

Munoz EC, Rosado JL, Lopez P, Furr HC, Allen LH (2000). Iron and zinc supplementation improves indicators of vitamin A status of Mexican preschoolers. Am J Clin Nutr 71: 789-94.

Muslimatun S, Schmidt MK, Schultink W, West CE, Hautvast JGAJ, Gross R, and Muhilal (2001). Weekly supplementation with iron and vitamin A during pregnancy increases haemoglobin concentration in Indonesian pregnant women. J Nutr; 131: 85-90.

Muslimatun S, Schmidt MK, West CE, Schultink W, Gross R, Hautvast JGAJ (2002). Determinants of weight and length of Indonesian neonates. Eur J Clin Nutr 56: 947-951.

Nail PA, Thomas MR, Eakin R (1980). The effect of thiamin and riboflavin supplementation on the level of those vitamins in human breast milk and urine. Am J Clin Nutr 33: 198-204.

Ndyomugyenyi R, Kabatereine N, Olsen A, Magnussen P (2008). Malaria and hookworm infections in relation to haemoglobin and serum ferritin levels in pregnancy in Masindi district, western Uganda. Trans Royal Soc Trop Med Hyg 102: 130-136.

Neggers YH, Cutter GR, Acton RT, Alvarez JO, Bonner JL, Goldenberg RL, Go RCP, Roseman JM (1990). A positive association between maternal serum zinc concentration and birth weight. Am J Clin Nutr 51: 678-84.

Neggers Y, Goldenberg RL (2003). Some thoughts on body mass index, micronutrient intakes and pregnancy outcome. J Nutr 133: 1737S-1740S.

Nhachi CFB, Kasilo OJ (1990). Occupational exposure to DDT among mosquito control sprayers. Bull Environ Contam Toxicol 45: 189-92.

Nobrega JA, Gelinas Y, Krushevska A, Barnes RM (1997). Direct determination of major and trace elements in milk by inductively coupled plasma atomic emission and mass spectrometry. JAAS 12: 1243-1246.

Nosten F, ter Kuile F, Maelankirri L, Decludt B, White NJ (1991). Malaria during pregnancy in an area of unstable endemicity. Trans R Soc Trop Med Hyg 85: 424-29

Nosten F, van Vugt M, Price R, Luxemburger C, Thway KL, Brockman A, McGready R, ter Kuile F, Looareesuwan S, White NJ (2000). Effects of artesunate-mefloquine combination on incidence of Plasmodium falciparum malaria and mefloquine resistence in western Thailand: a prospective study. Lancet 356: 297-302.

O'Brien KO, Zavaleta N, Caulfiled LE, Wen J, Abrams SA (2000). Prenatal iron supplements impair zinc absorption in pregnant Peruvian women. J Nutr 130: 2251-5.

Oostenburg GS, Mensink RP, Al MDM, van Houwelingen AC, Hornstra G (1998). Maternal and neonatal plasma antioxidant levels in normal pregnancy, and the relationship with fatty acid unsaturation. Br J Nutr 80: 67-73.

Ortega RM; Andres P, Martinez RM, Lopez-Sobaler AM, Quintas ME (1997). Zinc levels in maternal milk: the influence of nutritional status with respect during the third trimester of pregnancy. Eur J Clin Nutr 51: 253-258.

Ortega RM, Lopez-Sobaler AM, Andres P, Martinez RM, Quintas ME, Requejo AM (1999). Maternal vitamin E status during the third trimester of pregnancy in spanish women: influence on breast milk vitamin E concentration. Nutr Res 19(1): 25-36.

Ortega RM, Martinez RM, Andres O, Marin-Arias L, Lopez-Sobaler AM (2004). Thiamin status during the third trimester of pregnancy and its influence on thiamin concentrations in transition and mature milk. Br J Nutr 92: 129-135.

Osrin D, Vaidya A, Shrestha Y, Baniya RB, Manandhar DS, Adhikaqri RK, Filteau S, Tomkins A, de L Costello AM (2005). Effects of antenatal multiple micronutrient supplementation on birth weight and gestational duration in Nepal: double-blind, randomised controlled trial. Lancet 365: 955-62.

Pamuk ER, Byers T, Coates RJ, Vann JW, Sowell AL, Gunter EW, Glass D (1994). Effect of smoking on serum nutrient concentrations in African-American women. Am J Clin Nutr 59: 891-5.

Panpanich R, Vitsupakorn K, Harper G, Brabin B (2002). Serum and breast milk vitamin A in women during lactation in rural Chiang Mai, Thailand. Ann Trop Pediatrics 22: 321-4.

Papathakis PC, Rollins NC, Chantry CJ, Bennish ML, Brown KH (2007). Micronutrient status during lactation in HIV-infected and HIV-uninfected South African women during the first 6 mo after delivery. Am J Clin Nutr 85: 182-92

Pathak P, Kapoor SK, Kapil U, Joshi YK, Dwivedi SN (2002). Copper nutriture amongst pregnant women in a rural area of India. Eastern Journal of Medicine 8 (1): 15-17.

Piammongkol S, Chongsuvivatwong V, Williams G, Pornpatkul M (2006). The prevalence and determinants of iron deficiency in rural Thai-Muslim pregnant women in Pattani Province. Southeast Asian J Trop Med Public Health 37(3): 553-8.

Prapamontol T and Stevenson D (1991). Rapid method for the determination of organochlorine pesticides in milk. J Chromatograph 552:249-257.

Prapamontol T, Rugpao S, Silprasert A, Yutabootr Y, Tubtong V, Wongtrakul J, Amatayakul K (1995). A geographic distribution of DDT and its metabolites in maternal sera from Chiang Mai. Proc Tri-University Joint Seminar & Symposium (Oct. 24-27,1995), CMU: 91-96.

Prentice AM, Roberts SB, Prentice A, Paul AA, Watkinson M, Watkinson AA, Whitehead RG (1983). Dietary supplementation of lactating Gambian women. Effect on breast-milk volume and quantity. Hum Nutr Clin Nutr 37: 53-64.

Prinzo ZW, De Benoist B (2002). Meeting the challenges of micronutrient deficiencies in emergency-affected populations. Proc Nutr Soc 61: 251-257.

Rajalakshmi K, Srikantia SG (1980). Copper, zinc and magnesium content of breast milk of Indian women. Am J Clin Nutr 33: 664-669.

Ramakrishnan U, Manjrekar R, Rivera J, Gonzales-Cossio T, Martorell R (1999). Micronutrients and pregnancy outcome: a review of the literature. Nutrition Research 19: 103-159.

Rasmussen KM (2001). Is there a causal relationship between iron deficiency or iron-deficiency anemia and weight at birth, length of gestation and perinatal mortality. J Nutr 131 (suppl): 590S-603S.

Reichart PA, Schmidt-Westhausen A, Theetranont C. Oral cancer in Northern Thailand. Experimental Pathology 1990; 40:229-231.

Riedel AE, Menefee A (1997). Assessment of nutrient adequacy of rations for displaced persons from Burma on the western border of Thailand. Bangkok, Thailand: Nutrition Incorporated; 1997.

Rindi G, Patrini C, Poloni M (1981). Monophosphate, the only phosphoric ester of thiamin in the cerebrospinal fluid. Cellular and Molecular Life Sciences (CMLS) 37 (9): 975-76.

Roberfroid D, Huybregts L, Lanou H, Henry MC, Meda N, Menten J and Kolsteren P (2008). Effects of a maternal multiple micronutrient supplementation on fetal growth: a double-blind randomized controlled trial in rural Burkina Faso. Am J Clin Nutr 88: 1330-40.

Roberts DR, Manguin S, Mouchet J (2000). DDT house spraying and re-emerging malaria. Lancet 356: 330-32.

Rogan W, Chen A (2005). Health risks and benefits of bis(4-chlorophenyl)-1,1,1-trichloroethane (DDT). Lancet 366: 763-73.

Roidt L, White E, Goodman GE, Wahl PW, Omenn GS, Rollins B, Karkeck JM (1988). Association of food frequency questionnaire estimates of vitamin A intake with serum vitamin A levels. Am J Epidemiology 128(3): 645-653.

Romieu I, Hernandez-Avilla M, Lazcano-Ponce E, Weber JP, Dewailly E (2000). Breast cancer, lactationhistory, and serum organochlorines. Am J Epidemiol 152(4): 363-370.

Rylander L, Nilsson-Ehle P, Hagmar L (2006). A simplified precise method for adjusting serum levels of persistent organohalogen pollutants to total serum lipids. Chemosphere 62(3): 333-6.

Sakurai T, Furukawa M, Asoh M, Kanno T, Kojima T, Yonekubo A (2005). Fat soluble and water-soluble vitamin contents of breast milk from Japanese women. J Nutr Sci Vitaminol 51(4): 239-47.

Salimi S, Yaghmaei M, Joshaghani HR, Mansourian AR (2004). Study of zinc deficiency in pregnant women. Iranian J Publ Health 33(3): 15-18.

Sanchaisuriya K, Fucharoen S, Ratanasiri T, Sanchaisuriya P, Fucharoen G, Dietz E, Schelp FP (2006). Thalassemia and hemoglobinopathies rather than iron deficiency are major causes of pregnancy-related anemia in northeast Thailand. Blood Cells Mol Dis 37(1): 8-11.

Sauberlich HE (1999). Laboratory tests for the assessment of nutritional status. Boca Raton, 2nd ed. New York, CRC press, 1999.

Scaife AR, McNeill G, Campbell DM, Martindale S, Devereux G, Seaton A (2006). Maternal intake of antioxidant vitamins in pregnancy in relation to maternal and fetal plasma levels at delivery. Br J Nutr 95: 771-778.

Scanlon KS, Yip R, Schieve LA, Cogswell ME (2000). High and low hemoglobin levels during pregnancy: differential risks for preterm birth and small for gestational age. Obstet Gynecol 96: 741-8.

Scarcinelli P, Pereira ACS, Mesquita SA, Oliveira-Silva JJ, Meyer A, Menezes MAC, Alves SR, Mattos R, Moreira JC, Wolff M (2003). Dietary and reproductive determinants of plasma organochlorine levels in pregnant women in Rio de Janeiro. Environ Res 91: 143-150.

Scholl TO (1998). High third-trimester ferritin concentration: associations with very preterm delivery, infection, and maternal nutritional status. Obstet Gynecol 92(2): 161-166.

Scholl TO, Chen X, Sims M, Stein TP (2006). Vitamin E: maternal concentrations are associated with fetal growth. Am J Clin Nutr 84: 14442-8.

Schrijver J, Speek AJ, Klosse JA, van Rijn HJM, Schreurs WH (1982). A reliable semi-automated method for the determination of total thiamine in whole blood by the thiochrome method with high performance liquid chromatography. Ann Clin Biochem 19: 52-56.

Schulpis KH, Karakonstantakis T, Gavrili S, Chronopoulou G, Karikas GA, Vlachos G and Papassotiriou I (2004). Maternal-neonatal serum selenium and copper levels in Greeks and Albaniens. Eur J Clin Nutr 58: 1314-1318.

Schweigert FJ, Bathe K, Chen F, Büscher U, Dudenhausen JW (2004). Effect of the stage of lactation in humans on carotenoid levels in milk, blood plasma and plasma lipoprotein fractions. Eur J Nutr 43: 39-44.

Semba RD, Muhilal, West KP Jr, et al. (2000). Hyporetinolemia and acute phase proteins in children with and without xerophthalmia. Am J Clin Nutr 72: 146-153.

Seshadri S (2001). Prevalence of micronutrient deficiency particularly of iron, zinc and folic acid in pregnant women in South East Asia. Br J Nutr 85 (suppl 2): S87-S92.

Sinha R, Patterson BH, Mangels AR, Levander OA, Gibson T, Taylor PR, Block G (1993). Determinants of plasma vitamin E in healthy males. Cancer Epidemiology, Biomarkers & Prevention 2: 473-479.

Siddiqui MKJ, Srivastava S, Srivastava SP, Mehrotra PK, Mathur N, Tandon I (2003). Persistent chlorinated pesticides and intra-uterine foetal growth retardation: a possible association. Int Arch Occup Environ Health 76: 75-80.

Skikne BS, Flowers CH, Cook JD (1990). Serum transferrin receptor. A quantitative measure of tissue iron deficiency. Blood 75 (9): 1870-76.

Slorach SA, Vaz R (1983). Assessment of human exposure to selected organochlorine compounds through biological monitoring. Swedish National Food Administration; ISBN 91-7714-004-4.

Sommerburg O, Zang Lun-Yi, van Kuijk FJGM (1997). Simultaneous detection of carotenoids and vitamin E in human plasma, J Chromatography B 695: 209-215.

Solomons NW. Competitive interaction of iron and zinc in the diet (1986). Consequences for human nutrition. J Nutr 116: 337-49.

Steer P, Alam MA, Wadworth J, Welch A (1995). Relation between maternal haemoglobin concentration and birth weight in different ethnic groups. BMJ 310: 489-491.

Steer PJ (2000). Maternal haemoglobin concentrations and birth weight. Am J Clin Nutr 71 (suppl): 1285S-7S.

Steurer A, Rosenbaum P, Heller WD, Scherer G, Sennewald E, Funk B, Schmidt W (1999). Effect of smoking and antioxidant vitamin concentrations of pregnant patients on birth weight of newborn infants. Z Geburtshilfe Neonatal 203(3): 110-4.

Strobel M, Tinz J, Biesalski HK (2007). The importance of β-carotene as a source for vitamin A with special regard to pregnant and breastfeeding women. Eur J Nutr 46 (suppl 1): 1-20

Stuetz W, Prapamontol T, Erhardt JG, Classen HG (2001). Organochlorine pesticide residues in human milk of a Hmong hill tribe living in Northern Thailand. Sci Total Environ 273: 53-60.

Stuetz W, McGready R, Thein Cho, Prapamontol T, Biesalski HK, Stepniewska K, Nosten F (2006). Relation of DDT residues to plasma retinol, α-tocopherol, and β-carotene during pregnancy and malaria infection: a case-control study in Karen women in Northern Thailand. Sci Total Environ 363(1-3): 78-86.

Suharno D, West CE, Muhilal, Logman M, de Waart FG, Karyadi D, Hautvast J (1992). Cross-sectional study on the iron and vitamin A status of pregnant women in West Java, Indonesia. Am J Clin Nutr 56: 988-93.

Suharno D, West CE, Muhilal, Karyadi D, Hautvast JG (1993). Supplementation with vitamin A and iron for nutritional anemia in pregnant women in west Java, Indonesia. Lancet 342: 1325-1328.

Sukrat B, Sirichotiyakul S (2006). The prevalence and causes of anemia during pregnancy in Maharaj Nakorn Chiang Mai Hospital. J Med Assoc Thai 89 Suppl. 4: S142-S145.

Suzuki K, Tanaka T, Kondo N, Minai J, Sato M, Yamagata Z (2008). Is maternal smoking during early pregnancy a risk factor for all low birth weight infants? J Epidemiol 18(3): 89-96.

Takimoto H, Yokoyama T, Yoshiike N, Fukuoka H (2005). Increase in low-birth-weight infants in Japan and associated risk factors, 1980-2000.

Tallaksen CME, Böhmer T, Bell H (1991). Concomitant determination of thiamine and its phosphate esters in human blood and serum by high-performance liquid chromatography. J Chromatography 564: 127-136.

Tamura T, Goldenberg RL, Johnston KE, DuBard M (2000). Maternal plasma zinc concentrations and pregnancy outcome. Am J Clin Nutr 71: 109-13.

Tanumihardjo SA (2002). Vitamin A and iron status are improved by vitamin A and iron supplementation in pregnant Indonesian women. J Nutr 132: 1909-1912.

TBBC, Thailand Burmese Border Consortium (2006). Programme Report for January to June 2006. (www.tbbc.org)

Teucher B, Olivares M, Cori H (2004). Enhencers of iron absorption: ascorbic acid and other organic acids. Int J Vitamin Nutr Res 74(6): 403-19.

Thurnham DI, Davies JA, Crump BJ, Situnayake AD, Davis M (1986). The use of different lipids to express serum tocopherol-lipid ratios for the measurement of vitamin E status. Annals of Clinical Biochemistry 23: 514-520.

Thuy PV, Berger J, Davidsson L, Khan NC, Lam NT, Cook JD, Hurrell RF, Khoi HH (2003). Regular consumption of NaFeEDTA-fortified fish sauce improves iron status and reduces the prevalence of anemia in anemic Vietnamese women. Am J Clin Nutr 78(2): 284-90.

Toole MJ (1992). Micronutrient deficiencies in refugees. Lancet 339: 1214-1216.

Traber MG (2007). Vitamin E regulatory mechanisms. Annu Rev Nutr 27: 347-362.

Tren R, Bate R (2001). Malaria and the DDT story. The Institute of Economic Affairs, London, 2001; ISBN 0 255 364997.

Turusov V, Rakitsky V, Tomatis L (2002). Dichlorodiphenyltrichloroethane (DDT): ubiquity, persistence, and risks. Environ Health Perspect 110 (2): 125-8.

Von Mandach U, Huch R, Huch A (1994). Maternal and cord serum vitamin E levels in normal and abnormal pregnancy. Int J Vitam Nutr Res 64: 26-32.

Vimokesant SL, Hilker DM, Nakornchai S, Rungruangsak K, Dhanamitta S (1975). Effects of betel nut and fermented fish on the thiamin status of northeastern Thais. Am J Clin Nutr 28: 1458-63.

Wang YP, Walsh SW, Guo JD & Zhang JY (1991). Maternal levels of prostacyclin, thromboxane, vitamin E, and lipid peroxides throughout normal pregnancy. Am J Obstetrics and Gynecology 165: 1690-1694.

Watson-Jones D, Weiss HA, Changalucha JM, Todd J, Gumodoka B, Bulmer J, Balira R, Ross D, Mugeye K, Hayes R, Mabey D (2007). Adverse birth outcomes in United Republic of Tanzania - impact and prevention of maternal risk factors. Bull World Health Organ 85: 9-18

Weissmann G (2006). DDT is back: let us spray! FASEB 20: 2427-2429.

WHO (1995). Maternal anthropometry and pregnancy outcomes. A WHO collaborative study. Bull World Health Organ 73 (suppl): 1-98.

WHO (1996). Indicators for assessing vitamin A deficiency and their application in monitoring and evaluating intervention programmes. Geneva, World Health Organization, 1996 (WHO/NUT/96.10).

WHO (1999). Thiamine deficiency and its prevention and control in major emergencies (WHO/NHD/99.13). WHO, Geneva, 1999.

WHO (2001). Iron deficiency anaemia: assessment, prevention, and control. WHO, Geneva, 2001.

WHO Expert Consultation (2004). Appropriate body-mass index for Asian population and its implication for policy and intervention strategies. Lancet 363(9403): 157-63.

WHO (2006). Indoor residual spraying: Use of indoor residual spraying for scaling up global malaria control and elimination. Geneva, World Health Organization, 2006 (WHO/HTM/MAL/2006.1112).

WHO (2007). The use of DDT in malaria vector control. WHO position statement, Geneva, World Health Organization, 2007.

Wielders JPM, Mink CJK (1983). Quantitative analysis of total thiamine in human blood, milk, and cerebrospinal fluid by reversed-phase ion-performance liquid chromatography. J Chromatogr 277: 145-56.

Wondmikun Y (2005). Lipid-soluble antioxidants status and some of its socio-economic determinants among pregnant Ethiopians at the third trimester. Public Health Nutr 8(6): 582-587.

Woodruff BA, Blank HM, Slutsker L, Cookson ST, Larson MK, Duffield A, Bhatia R (2006). Anemia, iron status and vitamin A deficiency among adolescent refugees in Kenya and Nepal. Public Health Nutrition 9(1): 26-34.

Xiao R, Sorensen TK, Frederick IO, El-Bastawissi A, King IB, Leisenring WM, Williams MA (2002). Maternal second-trimester serum ferritin concentrations and subsequent risk of preterm delivery. Paediatric and Perinatal Epidemiology 16: 297-304.

Yagi N, Kamohara K, Itokawa Y (1979). Thiamine deficiency induced by polychlorinated biphenyls (PCB) and dichloro diphenyl trichloroethane (DDT) administration to rats. J Environ Pathol Toxicol 2: 1119-25.

Yamini S, West KP Jr, Wu L, Dreyfuss ML, Yang DX, Khatry SK (2001). Circulating levels of retinol, tocopherol and carotenoid in Nepali pregnant and postpartum women following long-term β-carotene and vitamin A supplementation. Eur J Clin Nutr 55: 252-259.

Yanez L, Ortiz-Perez D, Batres LE, Borja-Aburto VH, Diaz-Ba F (2002). Levels of dichlorodiphenyltrichloroethane and deltamethrin in humans and environmental samples in malarious areas of Mexico. Environ Res Section A 88: 174-181.

Yang MS, Chang FT, Chen SS, Lee CH, Ko YC (1999). Betel quid chewing and risk of adverse pregnancy outcomes among aborigines in southern Taiwan. Public Health 113(4): 189-92.

Yang MS, Chung TC, Yang MJ, Hsu TY, Ko YC (2001). Betel quid chewing and risk of adverse birth outcomes among aborigines in eastern Taiwan. J Toxicol Environ Health A 64(6): 465-72.

Yip R (2000). Significance of an abnormally low or high hemoglobin concentration during pregnancy: special consideration of iron nutrition. Am J Clin Nutr 72: 272S-279S.

Zagre NM, Desplats G, Adou P, Mamadoultaibou A, Aquayo VM (2007). Prenatal multiple micronutrient supplementation has greater impact on birth weight than supplementation with iron and folic acid : a cluster-randomized, double-blind, controlled programmatic study in rural Niger. Food Nutr Bull 28(3): 317-27.

Zavaleta N, Caulfield LE, Garcia T (2000). Changes in iron status during pregnancy in Peruvian women receiving prenatal iron and folic acid supplements with or without zinc. Am J Clin Nutr 71: 956-61.

Ziari SA, Mireles VL, Cantu CG, Cervantes M, Idrisa A, Bobsom D, Tsin ATC, Glew RH (1996). Serum vitamin A, vitamin E, and beta carotene levels in pre-eclamptic women in northern Nigeria. Am J Perinatol 13(5): 287-291.

Acknowledgements

Many people were involved in the present study, and many scientists and friends both in Germany and Thailand supported me in the overall five years study period.

I would like to express my sincere gratitude to Prof. Hans-Konrad Biesalski, my supervisor in Hohenheim, for his support and the constructive discussions.

Special thanks go to Prof. François Nosten, the principle investigator of the study who became my supervisor in Thailand, for his encouragement and support throughout the whole work. My deepest gratefulness goes to Dr. Verena Carrara, Dr. Sue Lee, Dr. Rose McGready and their collegues from the Shoklo Malaria Research Unit in Mae Sot and the Tropical Medicine at the Mahidol Univerisity. Dear Verena, you had the hard job to inform me on background and details regarding operation in the SMRU clinics in Maela camp as well as to introduce me in epidemiology and statistics. Dear Sue, thanks a lot for your exceptional help in statistical analysis, your suggestions in data evaluation, and for being my teacher in statistics and 'modeling'. Dear Rose, I am very grateful for your critical review and the many helpful comments on the latest manuscript.

My particular thanks are due to Dr. Tippawan Prapamontol and the 'Pollution and Environmental Health Research Group' at the Research Institute for Health Sciences (RIHES) in Chiang Mai for the successful long-term collaboration respecting the analysis of DDT in blood and breast milk samples. The RIHES became my second home during the residences in Thailand and I still feel most welcome in the 'family'.

My deepest appreciation goes to my partner Sigrun, my son Sebastian and the whole family for their borne endurance regarding the yearly trips with several months of residences in Thailand and the time I spend in the lab and finally at home for data analysis and to write up the PhD thesis.

I want to express my gratitude to Prof. Donatus Nohr who always supported my work and to Michael Wolter for the many fruitful discussions and the help during establishing new lab methods at the Institute of Biological Chemistry and Nutrition in Hohenheim.

Special thanks go to Dr. Jürgen Erhardt for his support in the analysis of iron status and infection markers and to Bärbel Horn and Dr. Jörn Breuer from the State Institute for Agricultural Chemistry, University of Hohenheim, for the successful collaboration regarding the analysis of trace elements (zinc, copper, iron) in serum and breast milk samples.

The financial support of my research work is gratefully acknowledged. In 2005 and 2006, the Eiselen foundation in Ulm, Germany supported me in the 'early phase' with money for the travels and living expenses in Thailand as well as for consumables for the lab analysis in Hohenheim. The Wellcome Trust, Great Britain funded the biochemical measurements including analysis on iron, micronutrients and DDT of the cross-sectional surveys in 2004. Laboratory supplies for blood and milk sampling and laboratory analysis regarding the cross-sectional and follow-up study in 2006-2007 were supported by the UBS Optimus Foundation in Zuerich, Switzerland. I am very grateful for the PhD scholarship 'Landesgraduiertenstipendium', a grant of the province Baden-Württemberg which I received from June 2006 to November 2008.

Finally, this work would not have been possible without the pregnant and post partum women in Maela refugee camp who participated in the studies. I wish that results and important findings of the present study will flow back in order to improve the nutrition situation and health status of the mothers and their infants.